THE
Naturally
CLEAN
HOME

121 Safe and Easy
Herbal Formulas for
Nontoxic Cleansers

Karyn Siegel-Maier

STOREY
BOOKS

*The mission of Storey Communications
is to serve our customers by publishing practical information that
encourages personal independence
in harmony with the environment.*

Edited by Deborah Balmuth and Robin Catalano
Cover design by Meredith Maker
Cover photograph by Giles Prett
Text design and production by Susan Bernier and
    Jennifer Jepson Smith
Indexed by Peggy Holloway, Holloway Indexing Services

Copyright © 1999 by Karyn Siegel-Maier

The information in this book is true and complete to the best of our knowledge. All recommendations are made without guarantee on the part of the author or Storey Books. The author and publisher disclaim any liability in connection with the use of this information. For additional information please contact Storey Books, Schoolhouse Road, Pownal, Vermont 05261.

Storey books are available for special premium and promotional uses and for customized editions. For further information, please call Storey's Custom Publishing Department at 1-800-793-9396.

Printed in Canada by Webcom Limited
10 9 8 7 6 5 4 3 2

Library of Congress Cataloging-in-Publication Data

Siegel-Maier, Karyn, 1960-
    The naturally clean home : 121 safe and easy herbal formulas for
    nontoxic cleansers / Karyn Siegel-Maier.
        p.   cm.
    Includes bibliographical references and index.
    ISBN 1-58017-194-X (pbk. : alk. paper)
    1. House cleaning.   2. Household supplies.   I. Title.
TX324.S24   1999
    648'.5—dc21   99-35380
                                                               CIP

CONTENTS

DEDICATION

This book is dedicated to you, the reader, whose commitment to better living is my inspiration and reward for writing.

· · ● ● ·

ACKNOWLEDGMENTS

Many thanks go to my loving husband, Andy, whose faith in me never falters — even when mine does. To Aaron, Michael, and Andy Jr. I offer my heart and hugs for your cooperation and understanding during this project, aside from giving me yet another excellent reason for undertaking it.

I also wish to express my sincere gratitude to Deborah Balmuth and Robin Catalano for their confidence in this book and their guidance in making it the best it can be.

Finally, I thank the forces that gently direct me in spirit each day, for giving me the opportunity to return the favor.

CLEAN
AND LET
LIVE

If your household is anything like mine, your Sunday mornings probably include the typical array of housekeeping activities, including washing, mopping, and polishing. There are probably a half-dozen things you'd rather being doing, but in the end it feels great to know the house is sparkling clean and a good space to be in. But is it? The grime and germs may have been whisked away, but something more ominous may have been left in their place — hazardous wastes. As you will soon learn, herbs can provide you with cleaning products that are just as effective, safer, and considerably less expensive than the products you may be using now.

HOUSEHOLD HAZARDS

You're probably not very comfortable with thinking of your home as akin to a toxic dump site. But if you consider how hazardous wastes are defined, you'll get a different picture of the nature of the "ordinary" substances used every day in your home.

Basically, any substance that is poisonous, carcinogenic, corrosive, reactive, flammable, or in some other way injurious to animals or humans is considered hazardous. Just like industrial hazardous materials, household chemicals possess one or more of these characteristics and require special handling. The difference is that too often the health risks of common household products are inadequately communicated or expressed in vague terms.

What Are the Dangers?

While only one in five of the four million household chemicals created since 1915 have actually been tested for their adverse health effects on humans, there is a surprising amount of alarming information that underscores their negative impact. Consider the following statistics:

- Ninety percent of all accidental poisonings occur in the home. According to the Columbia College of Physicians and Surgeons, more than seven million cases of poisonings are reported each year. That equates to 14,000 each day! Young children are the primary victims, with the elderly being the next most affected.
- According to a five-year EPA study, the air in an average American home has chemical contamination levels 70 times greater than outdoor air. The EPA maintains that half of all illnesses occurring in the United States can be attributed to chemical contamination of indoor air. In fact, a 1985 EPA report states that household cleaners are three times more likely to cause cancer than outdoor air pollution.

■ A study by the Toronto Indoor Air Commission concluded that, due to increased exposure to household carcinogens, women who work at home have a 55 percent greater chance of developing cancer than women who spend the majority of their time outside the home.

■ The National Academy of Science estimates that 15 percent of all Americans are multi–chemically sensitive due to chronic exposure to household and cosmetic products.

■ In 1990 alone, more than 4,000 children under the age of four were given emergency treatment for poisoning by consumption of a household cleaner. In the same year, nearly 18,000 pesticide-related incidents were reported in which 74 percent of the victims were younger than 14 years of age.

■ The Consumer Product Safety Commission has determined that more than 150 chemicals found in ordinary household products are directly responsible for producing cancer, allergies, birth defects, and numerous psychological disorders.

■ Dr. Russell Jaffe of Serammune Physicians Lab in Reston, Virginia, studied the long-term effects of pesticides on humans. He believes that as many as 16 million people in the United States evidence some degree of adverse reaction due to constant exposure. Of this number, Dr. Jaffe estimates that for five million people the results are ultimately fatal, 11 million are plagued with muscle and joint pain, and 500,000 are afflicted with migraines, asthma, bronchitis, and eczema.

■ In December 1984, the *Los Angeles Times* reported that "adverse effects from [household] chemicals include reduced male sperm count, testicle atrophy and infertility." Several European studies in the early 1990s not only found that the sperm count of the human male has dropped by half since 1938, but that future generations are threatened as well. Prior to the boom of chemical industrialization, a healthy adult male produced millions of sperm per milliliter of semen, but this number is steadily declining. In 1975, the typical 30-year-old man measured an average of only 102 million sperm per milliliter. And in 1992? You guessed it — the average 30-year-old produced a mere 51 million sperm per milliliter. This trend is expected to continue.

■ For children under ten years of age living where home or garden pesticides are frequently used, the risk of leukemia increases by four to seven times. Childhood brain cancer is also associated with the use of flea collars, herbicides, pesticides that target termites, and pesticide "bombs" used indoors.

Environmental Impact

Are those seemingly harmless and gaily packaged cleaners stored under your kitchen sink starting to sound scary? If they can be so harmful to you and your family, it should be fairly obvious that their impact upon vegetation and wildlife is equally negative. Therefore, please refrain from the temptation to flush or toss them away; you'll be doing more harm than good in an attempt to "set things right."

You may rationalize that the small amount you'll be dumping has little effect on the "big picture." This kind of faulty thinking has created pollution on a global scale; in an average city, nearly 168 tons of household cleaners are released into kitchen and bathroom drains every year. In fact, the EPA characterizes the typical American household as "the number one violator of chemical waste per capita." Aside from the direct impact the chemicals have when introduced into the environment, there are other complications to consider when disposing of their containers.

The average person contributes 3.5 pounds of waste product per day to the whole garbage pie, a sobering increase of 90 percent from only 30 years ago, before the dawn of commercial manufacturing of household products. Many products are packaged in nonrecyclable containers. If all those containers aren't being collected with the recycling, where do they wind up? The answer, of course, is the landfill. During the last 20 years, more than 75 percent of our landfills have reached maximum capacity, and the EPA estimates that more than half of those remaining will be filled up over the next 20 years. Furthermore, a considerable portion of this waste is laden with residual chemicals that eventually seep into the soil, contaminating groundwater and surface runoff leading to lakes and streams.

The use and disposal of such products have very clear, far-reaching ramifications on both the earth and its inhabitants. We are slowly destroying our environment. We have also been manipulated into destroying ourselves in the process, just a little quicker.

HIDDEN DANGERS

The dangers of some household products, such as bleach and caustic drain cleaners, are obvious and well known. But others may be seemingly harmless, and yet they contain ingredients that are just as deadly. The following is a sampling of some common household cleaning products and the typical constituents that threaten harm. This list barely skims the surface of the toxin pool, but it gives you an idea of what you and your family are being exposed to every day.

Furniture Polish

These commonly used cleaners contain petroleum distillates, naphthas, nitrobenzene, phenol (carbolic acid), mineral spirits, diglycol laurate, amyl acetate, and petroleum-based waxes. Petroleum distillates are highly flammable and can damage skin and lung tissue. Mineral spirits, naphtha, diglycol laurate, and amyl acetate depress the central nervous system. Nitrobenzene is extremely toxic and readily absorbed through the skin. Phenol is also absorbed through the skin and can cause convulsions, coma, respiratory arrest, or possibly death. It is also a nerve-deadening agent that can inhibit your sense of smell. Diglycol laurate can cause damage to the liver and kidneys. Phenol, nitrobenzene, naphthas, and other petroleum distillates are classified as hazardous wastes.

Dishwashing Liquids

Would you believe that the bottle of dishwashing soap you probably keep on the corner of your sink contains harmful chemicals such as naphtha, phosphates, sodium nitrates, petroleum-based surfactants, diethanolamine, and chloro-ortho-phenylphenol? Naphtha is a neurotoxin and chloro-ortho-phenylphenol is highly toxic. Both are classified as hazardous wastes. In the environment, chloro-ortho-phenylphenol can form other compounds that are absorbed and retained in the fatty tissue of living organisms, a process known as bioconcentration. Diethanolamine is a caustic substance, suspected of being a liver poison. Petroleum products are nonrenewable resources that break down slowly in the environment and remain long-term pollutants, and phosphates promote the overgrowth of algae. Dishwashing liquid is a leading cause of accidental poisonings in small children.

Automatic Dishwasher Detergents

Phosphates, sodium silicates, and highly concentrated dry chlorine are all found in these frequently used products. Automatic dishwasher detergents are highly alkaline and can burn the mouth and hands of a curious toddler, or the esophagus if accidentally swallowed. Dishwasher detergent is a leading cause of fatal poisonings in small children.

Drain Cleaner

Not surprisingly, these super-strong cleaners are made up of sodium hydroxide (lye), sulfuric acid, hydrochloric acid, and trichloroethane. Lye is caustic and can seriously burn the skin and eyes, as well as the stomach and esophagus if swallowed. Hydrochloric acid is corrosive and can damage the kidneys and liver. Trichloroethane is an eye and skin irritant, a neurotoxin, and can also damage the kidneys and liver. Many drain crystals contain highly concentrated forms of lye, bleach, and ammonia.

Oven Cleaners

Lye, methylene chloride, 2-butoxyethanol, chlorine, potassium hydroxide, ammonia, and petroleum distillates are the toxic culprits in oven cleaners. Most of these ingredients are recognized as hazardous wastes. Methylene chloride can damage the liver and kidneys and is stored in the fatty tissue of living organisms. With the exception of lye, all of these agents suppress the central nervous system when inhaled and can precipitate respiratory failure. The dangers are compounded for those who suffer from asthma.

Disinfectants

These aggressively marketed liquids and powders have quite a list of harmful ingredients, including naphtha, 2-butoxyethanol, triclosan, phenol, formaldehyde, benzalkonium chloride, ethanol, and sodium sulfites. With an impressively toxic list such as this, one wonders which is less offensive — a few invading germs, or the solution that seeks to destroy them. "Destroy" is right on the mark, because that's what benzalkonium chloride does to mucous membranes. Phenols can cause liver and kidney damage and are also nerve-deadening agents. Sodium sulfites can be fatal to asthmatics. Triclosan is readily absorbed through the skin and is associated with liver damage.

Laundry Detergent

Prepare yourself for quite a list here, including ammonium compounds, tetrapotassium pyrophosphate, sodium toluene, sodium alkylbenzene sulfonate, fluosilicate, benzethonium chloride, optical brighteners, sodium tripolyphosphate, sodium or calcium hypochlorite, and ethylenediaminetetraacetic acid (EDTA). Alkylbenzene sulfonate is easily absorbed through the skin and is known to damage the liver. Tetrapotassium pyrophosphate is very toxic, and fluosilcate is actually a pesticide. Sodium hypochlorite (bleach) and calcium hypochlorite are both highly corrosive and can burn eyes, skin, and lungs. EDTA binds with heavy metals in waterways, creating an overload of toxic metals. Optical brighteners (additives that reflect light to make clothes appear cleaner and brighter) can trigger severe allergic reactions and facilitate mutation of certain bacteria.

Toilet Bowl Cleaners

In our efforts to keep the commode clean, we are exposing ourselves to hydrochloric acid, hypochlorite bleach, phenols, oxalic acid, para-dichlorobenzene (PDB), naphtha, o-Dichloro-benze, p-Dichlorobenze. Hydrochloric acid is highly corrosive. Hypochlorite bleach is also corrosive and can cause pulmonary edema or coma if ingested. Inhalation of dichlorobenze can damage the liver and kidneys. Most of these ingredients can be stored in fatty tissue of living organisms and are classified as hazardous wastes.

Mold & Mildew Cleaners

Are you taking a bath with sodium hypochlorite (bleach), sodium hydroxide (lye), ethanol, and formaldehyde? Then you should know that sodium hypochlorite and sodium hydroxide are corrosive and can burn the eyes, throat, skin, and lungs. Formaldehyde is highly toxic and considered a carcinogen. Ethanol can destroy mucous membranes.

Air Fresheners

These fresh-smelling sprays actually poison the environment with formaldehyde, naphthalene, p-Dichlorobenzene, phenol, sodium bisulfate, methoxychlor, piperonyl butoxide, and o-phenylphenol. Naphthalene and p-Dichlorobenzene suppress the central nervous system, while formaldehyde and piperonyl butoxide are known carcinogens. Methoxychlor is a pesticide and readily stored in the fatty tissue of living organisms. Even more frightening is the fact that many air fresheners are chemically engineered to coat the nasal passages with an oily film and/or a nerve-deadening agent to interfere with the sense of smell.

Carpet and Upholstery Shampoo

Trichloroethylene, naphthalene, ammonium hydroxide, and perchlorethylene (dry cleaning fluid) are the main toxins found in carpet and upholstery cleaners. Ammonium hydroxide is corrosive and damaging to skin, eyes, and lungs. Trichloroethylene can cause cardiac arrhythmia or respiratory arrest. Perchlorethylene is a known carcinogen and impairs the liver, kidneys, and nervous system. Both trichloroethylene and perchlorethylene enter the body through inhalation and are stored in fatty tissue.

PESTICIDES HARM MORE THAN PESTS

Exposure to pesticides deserves a discussion on its own due to their widespread use in homes and offices as well as in agriculture. Their toll on human (and animal) health is very frightening.

What Makes a Pesticide Harmful?

Dichlorobenzene, tetramethrin, diazinon, organophosphates, chlorinated hydrocarbons, copper naphthenate — this is only a small sampling of the potential ingredients of any given pesticide, and all are highly toxic. For instance, diazinon is extremely toxic and affects the central nervous system, while chlorinated hydrocarbons are suspected of being carcinogens and mutagens.

It is estimated that nearly three million pesticide-related accidents occur each year worldwide and result in the loss of approximately 220,000 lives. Statistics show that, after death or injury due to contact with household cleaning products, pesticides are the next most common cause of poisoning in young children.

But you don't have to ingest a pesticide or fall victim to a factory spill to be put in harm's way. If you live among the general population, you are exposed to constant low levels of pesticide constituents via residential and commercial spraying, garden insecticides, and residual amounts found in the environment. These agents are stored in the fatty tissue of humans and animals and are linked to a variety of cancers, diseases of the blood, mental and behavioral disorders, learning disabilities (such as attention deficit disorder), and chemical sensitivity. Even if all pesticides were done away with today, the genetic dispositions of successive generations would still continue to evidence their effects.

The Devastating Effects on Children

A nine-year study published in *Chemosphere* in 1998 analyzed the breast milk of 139 nursing women with infants suffering from a variety of disorders requiring hospitalization. High levels of

PCBs were found in all of the samples. For those mothers whose infants had neurological disorders, the samples revealed even higher levels. Recent German studies have also revealed an association between pesticide exposure (including flea collars) and a greater incidence of childhood leukemia and brain cancer.

Another study published the same year in *Environmental Health Perspectives* examined the effect of pesticides on children who live in the Yaqui Valley of northwestern Mexico. Since the late 1940s, pesticides have been used heavily in this agricultural region. In 1990 researchers discovered significant levels of several pesticides in breast milk and in the cord blood of newborns. In the 1998 study, it was found that when compared to children residing in the foothills of the valley, which is pesticide free, the exposed children demonstrated a lack of energy, limited gross and fine eye-hand coordination, short-term memory loss, and the inability to draw a human figure.

Children are especially susceptible to the risks of pesticides. Since their bodies and defense systems are underdeveloped, it takes less exposure to cause harm. Another factor to consider is that young children spend a good deal of time crawling around on the floor during play and have a particular talent for finding nooks and crevices an adult would never think of inspecting. But that's just the kind of place where residue from pesticide spraying is likely to be found. Imagine a toddler's small, curious fingers exploring such an area and then finding their way to eyes, nose, and mouth.

According to a paper published in *Environmental Health Perspectives* in June 1998, "Recent findings of indoor exposure studies of chlorpyrifos indicate that young children are at higher risks to the semivolatile pesticide than had been previously estimated." The study revealed that after a single application of the pesticide in an apartment building, the toxin in question continued to build up on indoor surfaces, including toys, for two weeks after spraying. The researchers further assert that, "the estimated chlorpyrifos exposure levels from indoor spraying for children are approximately 21 to 119 times above the current recommended reference dose of 3 micrograms per kilogram per day from all sources."

Pesticides and Prescription Drugs: Tom Latimer's Story

We are also in the dark about the dangers of being exposed to the combinations of chemicals found in pesticides and their potential to react with other agents, such as pharmaceutical medications. For Tom Latimer, two seemingly innocent and unrelated events — taking Tagamet to control excessive stomach acid and mowing his lawn — combined to change his life forever.

Tom's incredible and tragic story unfolded in a 1991 article published in the *Wall Street Journal*. In the weeks prior to the incident, Tom had made an application of an organophosphate to his lawn in order rid it of ants. One morning, he and his wife decided to do some yard work. After an hour, Tom was complaining of nausea and dizziness.

A week later he was afflicted with chronic headaches and involuntary jerking of his eye muscles. Upon extensive examination and interview, it was discovered that Tom had been taking Tagamet, which, like aspirin and other anti-inflammatory drugs, interferes with the liver's function of eliminating toxins from the body. Unable to adequately defend himself against the toxins in the pesticide, his nervous system fell under attack. Even though he was treated, Tom still suffers today; he has trouble walking and is forced to take an anti-epileptic medication to help control his movements.

The *Good* News

So what's the good news in all of this? You can take steps to help prevent you and your children from becoming victims. You may not be able to avoid PCBs and organophosphates entirely, but you can significantly reduce your exposure by not using or storing pesticides around the house and garden. If you notice signs posted in your neighborhood indicating that any grass or lawn has been sprayed with pesticides, don't walk on it, and keep children and pets away from such areas.

Try to buy organic produce whenever possible, since their surfaces are free of pesticide and wax residue. (Be warned, however, that even organic produce can hold contaminants because much of our soil yields plants that are systemic; that is, contaminated groundwater invades the surrounding soil and the vegetation absorbs the chemicals.) All produce should be washed with a vegetable brush and vegetable-based soap.

No one likes to share a home with insects or rodents. But you must remember that pesticides are designed to kill living things — *all* living things. There are alternatives to using these poisons that not only harm the environment, but can lead to tragedy for those you love. The formulas on page 50 will help you safely keep pests at bay.

WHERE ARE THE CHEMICAL COWBOYS?

By now you're probably thinking that if the products we buy and use every day are really that harmful, they wouldn't be on the market in the first place, right? Sadly, this belief is wrong. While watchdog agencies do exist, the truth is that a household product is only scrutinized in response to numerous complaints, possibly long after a product has been placed on the market.

There are certain criteria to be met of course, but the Consumer Product Safety Commission (an advocate agency formed under the Federal Hazardous Substances Act), as well as the EPA, are sometimes misled into accepting a chemical, or chemicals, as safe by being presented with falsified research. Both Industrial Bio-Test and Craven labs were found guilty of this maneuver in 1983 and 1992, respectively.

Furthermore, we live in a world that is literally saturated with synthetic and hazardous chemicals, too many to keep track of. Government agencies also must contend with chemical lobbyists who push for safe registration of chemicals in an "innocent until proven guilty" tactic. When it comes down to it, the chemical manufacturing industry is all about the business of money.

WHAT SHOULD WE DO?

To be fair, government agencies do try to protect us from harm, even though the loopholes for misinformation and secrecy on the part of manufacturers seem wide open. Unfortunately, these agencies also operate with limited time, money, and manpower. Evaluating a particular chemical prior to marketing can cost in excess of $300,000. It should also be said that some manufacturers have responded to the grassroots population and share a concern about the safety of their products. According to *Chemical Engineering News,* manufacturers spend an approximate average of $150 million on studies and public relations to persuade consumers that their products are safe.

If you're feeling at all guilty that you may have been exposing yourself and your loved ones to any number of potential health risks for years, let me just say that it isn't your fault. You haven't been lazy, irresponsible, or morally and socially negligent. You have, however, been manipulated, misinformed, and, in some cases, blatantly lied to. Our friends at the EPA have also been fooled, since more than 300 chemicals used in a variety of products have been registered as safe due to fraudulent, even fictitious test data since the 1980s. But now that you have been empowered with the facts, you can take command with your buying power.

Learn to Decipher Labels

Exactly what chemical agents are being added to cleaning products remains a mystery to most of us, partly because many formulas are treated as closely guarded trade secrets, and partly because of inadequate labeling standards.

You might be shocked to learn that manufacturers are not required to list specific ingredients on the labels of their products. To make matters worse, a study done by the New York Poison Control Center revealed that 85 percent of product labels carried insufficient warnings regarding immediate and long-term health risks. Manufacturers are also not required to list inert ingredients, even though they could comprise up to 99 percent of the product's composition. This means that you, the consumer, are left out of the loop, without access to reliable information that would help you make an informed decision about a product.

There are labeling standards in effect of course, but they are a bit tricky, at least for the consumer. Suppose you were to come across a product at your grocery store with a label containing the word "nontoxic." You could feel pretty good about tossing that one in your cart because it must be safe, right? Not necessarily. There is no federal regulatory definition of nontoxic. In reality, it is merely an advertising word.

There are other terms used on product labels that are vague or designed to misinform, such as "biodegradable." What exactly does the manufacturer mean when it claims the product to be biodegradable? A better question to ask is how long will it take to biodegrade? Plutonium, for instance, is definitely biodegradable, but in a span of a thousand years. Once again, the well-meaning shopper ends up comparing apples to oranges when it comes to understanding cleaning product labels.

The key to buying cleaning products off the shelf is to strive to find those with labels that state the product is *readily* biodegradable and made from natural, renewable sources such as plant extracts and oil-based soaps.

Take It Step by Step

You will soon discover that switching from buying commercial toxic cleaners to buying or preparing nontoxic formulas may take an adjustment, and a bit of time. First of all, there is the array of products already in your home that you must confront. The least helpful thing would be to dump the hazardous cleaners you have down the drain or to throw them in the trash. Instead, contact your local agencies — such as your town or city hall — and find out if there is a hazardous waste collection program in place.

Of course, you could also use up what products you have and stand firm not to replace them with more of the same. Depending on the product type and its degree of toxicity, it's your judgment call. With the all-natural cleaners you'll learn to make, eventually your supply of cleaning products will diminish in number from dozens down to a mere handful — and they will be perfectly safe for you, your family, and the environment.

WHY CLEAN WITH HERBS?

Nearly everyone has heard about the virtues of common items such as baking soda and vinegar for cleaning jobs like scouring and absorbing grease. The addition of herbal materials, especially essential oils, to the formula serves to enhance its cleaning value with the added benefit of leaving behind a soothing, natural scent. In effect, the principles of sanitary hygiene and aromatherapy become partners. It's not by advertising gimmick that many commercial products contain citrus oils, such as lemon or lime; they are natural degreasers and have antimicrobial properties. In fact, citrus oils are the "workhorses" of the kitchen and bathroom. Many other herbs possess antibacterial and antifungal qualities as well. The chart on pages 26–27 gives more information on the beneficial cleaning properties of specific herbs.

THE BENEFITS OF NATURAL CLEANING

You can believe me when I tell you that using a natural herbal product instead of a chemical-laden commercial one makes household tasks almost a pleasure to tackle. I know it's hard to get excited about cleaning a bathroom, but when you realize that the surfaces are germ and toxin free, and the soothing aroma of cedar or lavender lingers, you won't be able to suppress a smile of satisfaction. And the enthusiasm is contagious — even the kids will want to pitch in!

Save Time and Money

Making your own herbal cleaning products is not a time-consuming or expensive endeavor. In fact, quite the opposite is true. It only takes a minute or two to fill a spray bottle with vinegar and water and add a few drops of essential oil. Bingo — instant glass and appliance cleaner! Having done that, there's one less aisle to visit in the supermarket.

The majority of commercial cleaners are quite expensive. A typical spray or foam cleanser for the bathroom, for instance, can deprive you of $4.00 or more. An herbal alternative, on the other hand, will cost mere pennies to make. I buy pure essential oils for an average of $3.00 per half fluid ounce. Since I am only using between 5 and 30 drops of the oil (depending on the particular formula), that half-ounce bottle goes a very long way indeed. Other all-natural ingredients, such as vinegar, baking soda, water, and castile soap are also inexpensive.

Unclutter Your Cleaning Closet

You will also marvel at the amount of uncluttered space that becomes available in the area where you normally store cleaning supplies. According to Debra Lynn Dadd, author of *Non-Toxic and Natural,* the average kitchen is home to thirty or more commercial products, the laundry room six!

Many of the herbal formulas you will be making will be multipurpose, so the number of cleaning products you store will be greatly reduced. This is an immense help, especially to those of us with only a little bit of space under the sink or in a closet.

CREATIVE PACKAGING

Why shouldn't the containers used to store your herbal cleaners be as pleasant as their contents? In this area, you can really exercise the concept of recycling materials. Remember those commercial products you finished up on your way to nontoxic cleaning? Many of those containers can be washed and used a countless number of times for your herbal formulas.

Coffee tins with plastic lids are great for storing car and wood polishes. Those large plastic containers with sprinkle-type tops you get when you purchase dried herbs and spices in bulk are excellent for powdered cleansers. Glass containers work well too, of course, but you may want to stick with plastic if safety is a concern, especially if "little helpers" may be using them.

WHICH HERBS TO USE

The formulas in this book suggest combinations of dried herbs and essential oils. Herb substitutions are encouraged when necessitated. The chart on pages 26–27 can help you make your selection according to the desired cleaning action.

For the most part, essential oils are suitable for all-purpose cleaning, floor and furniture care, and laundry needs. Strong tinctures can be used in place of essential oils in some formulas, if necessary, but their cleaning power will be less effective if used in laundry recipes, or those intended to be antibacterial. For obvious reasons, dried herbal material won't do for these tasks, but are excellent for other jobs such as scouring tubs and sinks and for use in carpet fresheners.

Purchasing Essential Oils

Essential oils and dried herbs are readily available in health food stores and by mail order. See Resources for a listing of good mail-order suppliers that sell both. But before you make any purchase, you should know that there are differences between herbal oils. Make sure that you're buying a pure, undiluted essential oil and not one that has been diluted in a carrier oil. Aromatherapy oils are a dilution of one or more essential oils with a "carrier" oil, such as almond or jojoba, and are intended for massage work and making perfume, among other things.

There are even grade differences among pure essential oils, but this difference generally pertains to the quality of fragrance, and for the purpose of household cleaning it is insignificant. Price may vary considerably as well, depending on the plant, its availability, and the extraction process.

Your essential oils will come in either blue or brown glass bottles. If stored away from heat and direct light, some essential oils will retain their potency indefinitely. Citrus oils are an exception; they usually last for about one year. Oil bottles usually come with droppers already built into the cap. The built-in dropper is there for a reason: to help you measure out the oil easily and control the number of drops you use. Use only the amount of essential oil called for in a recipe. The oils are highly concentrated, and adding more won't make a "super" formula; instead, it can increase the risk of skin irritation.

Keep in mind that essential oils can irritate the skin and must be diluted with a "carrier" oil or other liquid before use. Always practice caution when handling essential oils, and never allow children to handle the pure oils. Wearing protective gloves is highly recommended if your skin will be coming into contact with the chosen cleaner.

Can I Make My Own Essential Oils?

The best quality essential oils are often made by steam distillation. Unless you're a complete naturalist with plenty of time on your hands, making essential oils at home can be costly and tedious. However, many herbal supply companies offer home "stills" in a variety of sizes and with a price range of $50 to more than $100. Either way, it still takes a hefty amount of plant material to extract a small vial full of essential oil. Personally, I find this idea impractical for my lifestyle and prefer to buy my oils.

Choosing the Oils to Use

Which essential oils do you need? I use a variety of oils in cleaning formulas simply because I enjoy many different scents and because I keep a varied supply on hand for other projects. You may decide to use only a handful, and that's fine. Here are the most common essentials oils called for in the formulas in this book:

- Cedar
- Citronella
- Eucalyptus
- Lavender
- Lemon
- Lime
- Mint (including peppermint, spearmint, and wintergreen)
- Pine
- Rosemary
- Sweet orange
- Tea tree

HERBS AND THEIR BENEFICIAL PROPERTIES

Many herbs have antibiotic, antiviral, antiseptic, and antifungal properties. The following list is not complete by any means, but it represents the most common herbs that are grown in home gardens and that are easily available in dried or essential-oil form.

Herb	Properties
Bay	antibacterial
Bergamot	antibiotic
Camphor	antibacterial
Cardamom	antibacterial
Chamomile	antibiotic, antibacterial
Cinnamon	antiviral
Citronella	antibacterial
Clove	antibiotic, antiviral
Cypress	antibacterial
Eucalyptus	antibiotic, antifungal, antiviral, antibacterial

Herb	Properties
Ginger	antibacterial
Hyssop	antibiotic, antibacterial
Juniper	antifungal, antibacterial
Lavender	antibiotic, antifungal, antiviral, antibacterial
Lemon	antibiotic, antifungal, antiviral, antibacterial
Lemongrass	antibacterial
Lemon verbena	antibacterial
Lime	antibiotic, antibacterial
Marjoram	antibacterial
Myrtle	antibiotic, antifungal
Nutmeg	antibiotic
Orange	antibacterial
Oregano	antibiotic, antiviral
Patchouli	antibiotic, antifungal
Pine	antibiotic, antibacterial
Rosemary	antibacterial
Sage	antifungal, antibacterial
Sandalwood	antifungal, antiviral, antibacterial
Savory	antifungal
Spearmint	antibacterial
Tea tree	antibiotic, antifungal, antiviral, antibacterial
Thyme	antibacterial, antifungal, antiviral, antibacterial
Vervain (also called verbena)	antibacterial
Wintergreen*	antibacterial

*Take extra care when handling

GROWING YOUR OWN HERBS

If you are fortunate enough to be able to grow your own herbs, as I do, you will already have a supply of herbal material on hand to dry for making scouring powders, sachets, and carpet fresheners. The dried flowers and leaves of many herbs — such as rosemary, sage, lavender, mint, and lemon balm — are suitable for these products. Most herbs are quite hardy, easy to grow, and add beauty to any lawn or garden. Let's not forget the contributions they make to meals!

You will need to dry the herbs before using them in cleaning formulas. The concentration of essential oils is highest just before and during flowering. You'll want to leave at least one-third of each perennial in the garden to ensure its return the following season.

Harvesting Herbs

The leaves and stems can be harvested by cutting into stalks just before or during flowering, when their essential oils are at their peak. Flowers can be used too, and they will be at their best at either the bud stage or in full bloom. Rose, lavender, and rosemary blossoms are all harvested this way, and are especially good additions to powdered cleansers.

Roots, rhizomes, and bulbs should be taken from biennials and perennials when their oils and nutrients are not being used for the plant's growth. This occurs during late summer or fall when the plant begins to die back and store nutrients underground for the winter, or in early spring as the first leaves begin to emerge. Ginger is a popular herb that is harvested in this manner.

Drying Herbs

The old-fashioned and most pleasant way to dry herbs is the method of air-drying. At the end of each summer, I cut several stalks of different herbs to hang in my kitchen to dry. The aroma is incredible! Unless you have a perfectly controlled climate, attics, basements, and garages are usually either too arid or too moist to dry herbs in. Moisture can cause molding, and you'll have to start over.

The key to air-drying successfully is to hang the herbs upside down in small bunches (four or five medium-size stalks each) and to provide a place where they will get sufficient air circulation and be sheltered from direct sunlight and extreme temperatures. Secure the stalks fairly tightly with string or ribbon; they shrink somewhat during the drying process and tend to slip away from the bunch. You don't want to find your herbs on the floor! You also might want to write the name of the plant on a small tag and attach it to the stalks. Unless you're familiar with herbs and their different scents, you might get confused about the identity of the dried product.

Ideally, herbs should hang freely from cup hooks or pegs to dry. No room in your kitchen? There's always the ceiling — they won't be in anyone's way up there. Special racks can be constructed or purchased for this purpose. Some people spread herbs out on screens to dry. This is fine, as long as you have the room and you do not expose the herbs to extreme heat or moisture.

In two to three weeks, the herbs should feel very dry and the leaves can then be stripped away from the stalk and crumbled into clean glass jars. Avoid storing dried herbs in plastic bags because the volatile oils of the herb will interact with the chemicals in the plastic.

Another method of drying herbs is in a food dehydrator. This is an excellent method because the plants dry evenly, as long as you don't pack the trays with too much material. Such quick drying preserves the essential oils, and you'll have the added benefit of dried herbs within a matter of hours instead of weeks. I bought my five-tier dehydrator at a garage sale a few years back. It was the best $2.00 I've ever spent. By the way . . . why not hang a few sprigs of herbs to air-dry in the kitchen anyway, just to capture the spirit of your craft? Their aroma will last for months and they lend a "homey" feel when on display.

I don't recommend drying herbs in the oven. Even at a low temperature setting, the herbs dry too quickly, their oils evaporate due to constant heat radiation, and they easily scorch.

Other Methods of Preserving Herbs

While drying is the most common and basic way to preserve herbs, there are several other methods you might wish to try due to space limitations or other concerns, such as a damp climate. The following are some of the more popular preservation techniques.

Infusions are like very strong teas. The herbal material, including flowers, is steeped in boiling water for at least 10 minutes, then strained and poured into clean containers. A general guide is one tablespoon of herb to each cup of water. Infusions can be used in a formula in place of water; rosemary, thyme, and oregano infusions are very helpful when used this way. When kept in the refrigerator, an infusion will last two to three weeks.

Decoctions are made to extract the essential oils from heavier materials, such as roots and bark. The herbal material is simmered for 10 to 30 minutes and the liquid then strained. Use about one ounce of herb to each cup water. Like infusions, decoctions can be stored in the refrigerator for up to three weeks. Gingerroot, cinnamon bark, and vanilla beans are examples of herbs that yield their beneficial properties when prepared in this way.

Tinctures, also called extracts, are a 1:1 solution of alcohol and water. (Vinegar is sometimes used in place of alcohol.) With this method, the herbal material is packed into a jar and completely covered with a solution of 50 percent alcohol (or vinegar) and 50 percent water and left to stand on a sunny shelf for two to three weeks. It helps to gently shake or turn the jar once a day to redistribute its contents. Tinctures may be used in cleaning formulas, but add only ½ ounce at a time. Because of the alcohol content, too much tincture in a formula can be irritating to both the lungs and skin.

Vinegars are made in the same manner as tinctures, but the vinegar is used full strength.

COMMON CLEANING TOXINS

There is no shortage of documentation to prove that many common household products are dangerous to the environment and your health. But there are several readily available all-natural alternatives that will make letting go of your familiar "standby" products painless. Some of these items you probably already have on hand. Other items can be found in most natural foods stores, hardware stores, and supermarkets.

A WORD ABOUT SAFETY

Although the ingredients you will be using to make cleaning formulas are of organic origin, that doesn't mean they are without consequences if ingested. Essential oils are highly concentrated forms of the volatile oils found in plants and should never be used internally. Just a few drops are equivalent to approximately 30 to 40 cups of herbal tea. Take special care with food-related oils; citrus oil, for example, could offer a temptation to a young child who may mistake a finished product or substance as something delicious to eat or drink. Essential oils, and other materials you find recommended in this book, can also be quite irritating to skin. Please exercise the same caution with your herbal cleaning formulas as you would any commercial cleaner, and keep them away from pets and children.

Soap vs. Detergent

Before the dawn of large-scale manufacturing, liquid soaps were made from saponins, foaming, sudsy substances found in the roots of soapwort, soapberry, and yucca. The typical liquid dishwashing soap bought from the grocery store is made from a petroleum distillate, a toxic pollutant and nonrenewable resource. This product is actually a detergent, not soap. The safe and natural alternative is a vegetable-based soap called *castile,* a pure soap made from coconut or olive oil. It is readily biodegradable and made from renewable sources.

Castile soap can be found in liquid or solid form in health food stores and, thankfully, some supermarkets. One of the best known brands (and my personal favorite) is Dr. Bronner's, which comes in concentrated form and often "pretreated" with herbal oils. The company also allots at least 10 percent of its profits to rain-forest preservation and homeless shelter support. Does the manufacturer of your commercial liquid detergent do the same?

The Dangers of Bleach

Bleach, or sodium hypochlorite, is a combination of chlorine and sodium hydroxide (caustic soda) and is perhaps one of the most difficult of commercial cleaning products to relinquish. Technically speaking, household bleach is not considered corrosive or toxic, even if ingested. It is however, classified as a skin and eye irritant. It can burn human tissue, internally or externally, especially in small children. In fact, the accidental swallowing of bleach is the most frequently received call at Poison Control Centers involving children under the age of six. But young, tender hands and lips can also suffer serious burns.

If household bleach can do such damage, and is so predominantly a factor in the accidental poisoning of young children, why keep it around the house? There are many natural and nontoxic solutions for removing stains and "keeping whites white." If you feel you must have access to a bottle of bleach, at least use one that is free of chlorine to reduce the risks. One of the best that I have used is made by Seventh Generation. Although the company doesn't supply its products on a retail level, they can often be found in health food stores and in some supermarkets. Treat this bleach as you would any other: store it in a locked cabinet or out of reach of pets and children.

GETTING STARTED

Now that you've decided to switch to all-natural cleaning products, you might be wondering what you need to get started. The following must-have items will create a large variety of cleaners for all sorts of different surfaces and jobs.

Supplies at a Glance

The basic supplies required for making your own cleaners are generally inexpensive and easy to find. To make the widest array of products for the home, the following are the items to have on hand.

■ **Baking soda.** Otherwise known as bicarbonate of soda, you can find this ingredient very inexpensively at any supermarket or grocery store, usually in the baking supplies aisle.

■ **Beeswax.** This solid substance, usually in chunk or brick form, is available at art and craft stores, candle supply shops, and sometimes from local beekeepers.

■ **Borax.** A combination of water, oxygen, sodium, and boron, borax is a powder sold in the laundry aisle of grocery stores. A popular brand is 20 Mule Team by the Dial Corporation.

■ **Carnauba wax.** The hardest natural wax known, made from a Brazilian palm tree, this item is sold by furniture stores and mail-order companies.

■ **Castile soap.** An important ingredient, liquid castile soap is sold at health food stores, some supermarkets, and via mail order.

■ **Citrus seed extract.** Usually made from grapefruit seed, this natural preservative is a powerful antimicrobial agent. It is often sold as grapefruit seed extract, and sometimes as liquid Paramycocidin, and is available through mail order, as well as at some health food stores.

■ **Cream of tartar.** A popular culinary ingredient, this powdered mixture is sold in a box in the herb and spice or baking aisle of any supermarket.

■ **Diatomaceous earth.** This powder, made from the skeletons of fossilized algae, is available at garden supply and hardware stores, as well as through mail-order companies. Note, however, that this type of diatomaceous earth is *not* the same substance that you can buy from pool supply centers.

■ **Essential oils.** These concentrated volatile oils of plants can be found at health food stores, specialty shops, and via mail order.

■ **Glycerin.** Glycerin is a useful liquid for cleaners, medicines, and even some craft projects. You'll find it at art and craft stores, some pharmacies, and natural food stores.

■ **Lanolin.** Lanolin, an oily substance derived from sheep's wool, can be purchased from mail-order companies.

■ **Murphy's Oil Soap.** A very popular liquid soap for wood, Murphy's is sold at just about any supermarket. Check the cleaning products aisle.

■ **White vinegar.** Used in many cuisines, white vinegar is found in the oil aisle of any supermarket.

Suggested Equipment

Many of these implements may already be on hand. Wash and rinse the containers from your old products and they're ready to service you again in your nontoxic cleaning chores. Be sure to label your product with a list of ingredients; any type of label from an office supply, stationery, or grocery store will do. While you're at it, be creative and give your formula a catchy name! Since labels can get wet, they are best covered with clear shipping tape or laminating sheets cut to size. Plan to keep the following around:

- Plastic squirt bottles of various sizes, depending on purpose
- Plastic spray bottles, small and large
- Plastic containers with shaker tops (spice containers are great)
- Misters (plastic pump spray bottles)
- Coffee cans with lids (great for storing waxes and pastes)
- Glass jars (preferably widemouthed) with screw-top lids
- Cotton cloths (to use instead of paper towels)
- Rags (T-shirts, scrap cotton cloth, old towels)
- Cellulose sponge cloth (made of natural cellulose, these are washable and durable)
- Gallon-size buckets for large jobs
- Mops (cotton head for floors, sponge head for carpets and walls)

KITCHEN

THE

To me, the kitchen is the hub and heart of a home. This room is more than a storage receptacle for culinary sundries; this is where we gather with cherished family and friends for mealtime celebrations. Unfortunately, this is also the room where the garbage is usually kept, where a bare floor endures the patter of muddy feet, and where the odor of grease and last night's fish stubbornly linger. In other words, it's a haven for germs. Save for the "loo," the kitchen is probably the most frequented room in the house and is most in need of daily cleaning.

It's a pity that most of us grew up to think a clean kitchen is only evidenced by the overwhelming and pungent smell of a pine solvent. And little did we realize that our nervous systems were being treated to an assault of toxins. But you can create your own cost-effective, healthy alternatives to all the kitchen cleaners you're accustomed to using.

WASHING THE DISHES

Dishwashing liquids and automatic dishwasher detergents have been designed to lure the consumer with their stimulating lemony scent. This is more than an advertising gimmick; sure, citrus oils smell nice, but they are also natural degreasers. It's the rest of the ingredients in these harsh detergents that we are better off without.

Dishwashing Liquids

The herbal essential oils recommended in the following formulas will pack a punch on germs and greasy dirt without knocking you out in the process.

SYNERGISTIC DISHWASHING BLEND #1

This fruity blend will have you looking forward to washing dishes!

>   liquid castile soap
>   15 drops lemon or lemongrass essential oil
>   6 drops lavender essential oil
>   5 drops bergamot essential oil

Fill a clean 22-ounce plastic squirt bottle with castile soap (diluted according to directions if using concentrate). Add the essential oils. Shake the bottle before each use. Add 1 to 2 tablespoons of the liquid to dishwater and wash as usual.

Synergistic Dishwashing Blend #2

Here's another sweet-smelling formula.

>   liquid castile soap
>   20 drops lime essential oil
>   10 drops sweet orange essential oil
>   5 drops citrus seed extract

Fill a clean 22-ounce plastic squirt bottle with castile soap (diluted according to directions if using concentrate). Add the essential oils. Shake the bottle before each use. Add 1 to 2 tablespoons of the liquid to dishwater and wash as usual.

Synergistic Dishwashing Blend #3

Enjoy the herbal fragrance as you wash!

>   liquid castile soap
>   10 drops lavender essential oil
>   8 drops rosemary essential oil
>   4 drops eucalyptus essential oil

Fill a clean 22-ounce plastic squirt bottle with castile soap (diluted according to directions if using concentrate). Add the essential oils. Shake the bottle before each use. Add 1 to 2 tablespoons of the liquid to dishwater and wash as usual.

Dishwashing Blues Blend

Try this recipe for an uplifting washing experience.

>   liquid castile soap
>   10 drops lemon essential oil
>   6 drops bergamot essential oil
>   4 drops lavender essential oil
>   2 drops orange essential oil

■ For very greasy dishes, add ½ cup vinegar or lemon juice to the dishwater.

■ To loosen baked-on food from pots and pans, immediately add some baking soda and wait 15 minutes before cleaning. If the pot or pan has cooled before you've had a chance to add baking soda, boil a solution of 1 cup water, 5 drops cedar or other essential oil, and 3 tablespoons baking soda directly in the pot or pan. Allow the mixture to stand until the food can be scraped off easily.

Fill a clean 22-ounce plastic squirt bottle with castile soap (diluted according to directions if using concentrate). Add the essential oils. Shake the bottle before each use. Add 1 to 2 tablespoons of the liquid to dishwater and wash as usual.

Automatic Dishwasher Detergents

In this department, there's good news and bad news. The bad news first: There aren't many materials available for making a dependable automatic dishwasher detergent that is effective, economically feasible, nontoxic, and readily biodegradable.

Now for the good news: There are several brands available in health food stores and some supermarkets that handle all of these concerns. Ecover, Life Tree, and Naturally Yours are brands that I have happily used and that can be found in health food stores. My local supermarket carries cleaners made by Earth Friendly Products, including a liquid automatic dishwasher detergent called Wave. Shaklee also makes one of my favorite automatic dishwasher detergents, a highly concentrated biodegradable powder.

OVEN CLEANERS

Commercial oven cleaners are one of the most toxic and unpleasant products you could use. If the fumes from the application aren't bad enough, the foul smell of chemical burn-off the stuff continues to produce is enough to make one afraid of turning on the oven! The following formulas work very well. No oven cleaner is a miracle worker, however. Sometimes it may require a bit of elbow grease if there's a great deal of buildup on your oven walls and floor.

When vinegar is added to baking soda a fizzing reaction occurs. While this might startle you at first, it is perfectly normal.

SUNDAY OVEN-CLEANING FORMULA

This formula is for regular oven maintenance.

> 2 tablespoons baking soda
> 2 tablespoons liquid castile soap
> 10 drops sweet orange, lemon, or lime essential oil
> ½ cup hot water

1. Preheat oven to 250°F for 15 minutes, then turn off and leave door open.
2. Combine the baking soda, soap, and essential oil in a clean spray bottle. Add the water and shake well.
3. Spray on oven walls and wait 20 minutes. Wipe clean and rinse well.

Serious Oven-Cleaning Formula

I once made a family-size turkey potpie in one of my best crocks and watched helplessly as it began bubbling over within minutes of putting it in the oven. What a mess! This formula is great for such disasters, or for ovens that have been neglected for a while.

 ½ cup salt
 ¼ cup washing soda or borax
 1 box (16 ounces) baking soda
 scant ¼ cup water
 ¾ cup white vinegar
 10 drops thyme essential oil
 10 drops lemon or lemongrass essential oil

1. Combine salt, washing soda, and baking soda in a plastic container or glass bowl. Add just enough water to make a paste.

2. Remove oven racks and preheat the oven to 250°F for 15 minutes, then turn off the oven and leave the door open. Carefully spread the paste on oven walls with a sponge or cloth and allow to set for 20 to 30 minutes.

3. Combine the vinegar and essential oils in a spray bottle and shake well. Spray the oven walls and wipe clean. Rinse well.

Note: If you have a lot of baked-on grease or food splatters, you may want to use fine steel wool to scrub those areas. Use a bit more salt if necessary.

OVERNIGHT OVEN CLEANER

Bring out these proven grease-cutting oils for those heavy-duty oven-cleaning jobs.

> 1 cup water, divided
> 10 drops sweet orange, lemon, or rosemary essential oil
> ½ cup salt, divided
> 1¼ cups baking soda, divided
> 2 teaspoons liquid castile soap
> ¼ cup vinegar

1. Block the vents in the oven floor with aluminum foil or waxed paper. Preheat oven to 300°F for 15 minutes, then turn off the oven and leave the door open.

2. Combine ¼ cup water with essential oil in a spray bottle and shake well. Spray oven floor and walls with this precleaning mixture.

3. Combine ¼ cup salt and ½ cup baking soda. Sprinkle the mixture on oven floor, paying particular attention to spill areas.

4. Mix ¼ cup water with the remaining ¾ cup baking soda, ¼ cup salt, and the castile soap. Spread this mixture on the oven walls. Remove the foil or waxed paper from the vents and allow the paste to sit overnight.

5. Combine the remaining ½ cup water with the vinegar in a spray bottle. In the morning, spray the oven walls and floor generously with this mixture. Wipe well, using fine steel wool to work off any stubborn spots. Rinse several times to remove any residue.

SOAK THOSE STOVE ACCESSORIES!

The chrome rings that surround burners on an electric stove, the grills that rest on gas stove burners, and oven knobs all collect grease and food splatters over time. While cleaning your oven, these items can soak in a solution of 1 cup baking soda, ½ cup vinegar, and 4 to 6 drops essential oil of your choice. Use a fine steel wool pad or old toothbrush to remove grime from small spaces.

THE KITCHEN SINK

The baking soda-essential oil mixtures in the following formulas can be made in larger batches and stored in a plastic container, glass jar, or coffee can (store the vinegar separately). I find the large plastic spice and herb jars with shaker tops are perfect for powdered cleaners. Just soak off the label and wash and dry the inside of the container.

BASIC SINK CLEANSER

This formula is safe for porcelain or stainless steel sinks. Not only will it clean the sink basin and faucets, but it will also keep drains and garbage disposals fresh-smelling and free of clogs. Note: A vinegar rinse can be used before the final hot water rinse to prevent residue from the baking soda.

>   ¼ cup baking soda
>   ½ cup vinegar
>   3 drops lavender, rosemary, lemon, lime, or
>   orange essential oil

Combine all ingredients. Rinse sink well with hot water. Pour the cleanser in the sink and wipe with a sponge or cloth. Rinse again with hot water.

Herbal Scrubber

You can make up this formula in larger batches and store it in an airtight container. Use only whole dried (not powdered) plant material for this recipe.

> ½ cup baking soda
> ½ cup dried sage leaves, coarsely ground
> ¼ cup rosemary leaves, ground

Combine the ingredients in an airtight container and shake well to blend. Sprinkle a small amount of the powder into the sink and scrub with a damp sponge. Rinse well.

Country Spice Scrubber

Simple and sweet!

> 1 cup baking soda
> 3 teaspoons ground cinnamon
> 3 drops cedar or sweet orange essential oil

Combine the ingredients in an airtight container and shake well to blend. Sprinkle a small amount of the powder into the sink and scrub with a damp sponge. Rinse well.

Sink Scrubber for Stains

For stubborn stains, allow this formula to rest on the stain for several minutes. Then scrub and rinse with vinegar and hot water.

> ¼ cup borax
> ¼ cup baking soda
> 8 drops rosemary, eucalyptus, or tea tree essential oil
> ¾ cup vinegar for rinsing

Combine the borax, baking soda, and essential oil in an airtight container and shake well to blend. Sprinkle a small amount of the powder into the sink and scrub with a damp sponge. Rinse sink with vinegar, then with hot water.

PORCELAIN SINK SAVER

If you have an old-fashioned porcelain sink in your kitchen then you know that even though they look lovely, they do take on scuff marks and stains rather easily. Try this herbal remedy for really stubborn spots.

> 1 part sage, rosemary, lemon balm, thyme, or mint, fresh or dried
> 1 part water

Brew a strong infusion by steeping the herb in hot water for 2 to 3 hours. Strain, reserving the liquid.

Close the sink drain, pour in the liquid, and allow it to work for several hours or overnight.

Note: If the stain persists, place 4 to 6 drops of your favorite essential oil directly on the stain for a few minutes and then scrub the spot with baking soda sprinkled on a damp sponge.

CLEANING FAUCETS

The best thing for cleaning faucets is a simple mixture of equal parts water and vinegar. If you have a buildup of grime around the base of the faucet, put 3 or 4 drops of a citrus essential oil directly on the dirt, then clean with a toothbrush.

SIMPLE SINK CLEANSER

Bon Ami brand cleanser is made of grated detergent and feldspar and is nontoxic and nonabrasive. Sprinkle it freely in the sink basin and add 5 or 6 drops essential oil of choice, if desired. Scrub and rinse well.

RUST REMOVER

Wipe away these unattractive stains with a fresh-scented cleaner. Note: If the stain is on the side of your sink, use more baking soda to make a thick paste that will cling to the spot.

> ¼ cup baking soda
> 5 drops essential oil of choice
> juice of half a lemon

Sprinkle baking soda directly on the rust stain. Add essential oil and sprinkle with lemon juice. Allow the mixture to sit on the stain undisturbed for several hours or overnight. Wipe away baking soda and rinse thoroughly.

CLEANING KITCHEN APPLIANCES

Kitchen appliances, such as refrigerators, microwave ovens, and dishwashers, can get grimy from cooking grease and odors. Let's not forget those little fingerprints! The following formulas will clean the appliances without scratching surfaces, and can be made in larger batches and stored in plastic spray bottles.

LEMON BLAST APPLIANCE CLEANER

This solution is great for refrigerators and stove tops.

> 1 teaspoon liquid castile soap
> ⅛ cup white vinegar
> ¼ cup lemon juice
> 2 cups water
> 6 drops citrus seed extract
> 4 drops lemon, lime, orange, or eucalyptus essential oil
> 1 teaspoon borax

Combine all ingredients in a plastic spray bottle. Shake well before each use. Spray generously on appliance surface and wipe with a damp cloth or sponge. Wipe dry with a cloth or towel.

HERBAL APPLIANCE DEGREASER

This formula will remove greasy film from appliance surfaces.

> 2 cups water
> ¼ cup oil-based soap (Murphy's is good)
> 10 drops rosemary, lavender, or citrus essential oil

Combine all ingredients in a plastic spray bottle. Shake well before each use. Spray generously on appliance surface and wipe with a damp cloth or sponge. Wipe dry with a cloth or towel.

CONTROLLING PESTS
IN THE KITCHEN

Here are some tips for keeping unwanted critters at bay:

Ants will be dissuaded if you wipe out your kitchen cabinets with a damp sponge and 6 to 8 drops of peppermint or citronella essential oil. Then place 3 to 5 drops of those essential oils on windowsills, doorway cracks, the edges where countertops meet the wall, and in the corners of the cabinet under your kitchen sink.

Centipedes, earwigs, and silverfish can be deterred by placing several drops of peppermint, wintergreen, eucalyptus, or citronella essential oil in areas that collect moisture, such as damp basements, garages, and cabinets that house plumbing fixtures.

Cockroaches, unfortunately, are very tough. You can sprinkle a mixture of borax and sugar in the dark areas where roaches like to hide, but this method might not be feasible if you have young children or pets. It may be best to consult an exterminator.

Insects in general can be deterred by loose bay leaves placed in your kitchen cabinets.

Mice dislike peppermint, so place several sprigs of fresh peppermint between pantry items in your cabinets. You can also make a solution of 2 cups water and 3 teaspoons of peppermint essential oil and spray it wherever you find mouse droppings.

Mites and **weevils** are repelled by a few whole nutmegs placed in flour bins or bags.

MICROWAVE CLEANER

The interior of a microwave oven can trap grease and cooking odors that can spoil the flavor of foods during cooking. Try this remedy whenever you think your microwave could use a little sprucing up. If your microwave has a glass turntable, remove it and wash by hand.

> ¼ cup baking soda
> 1 teaspoon vinegar
> 5–6 drops thyme, lemongrass, or lemon essential oil

Combine all ingredients to make a paste. Apply to the walls and floor of the microwave with a soft cloth or sponge. Rinse well and leave the microwave door open to air-dry for about 25 minutes.

REFRIGERATOR & FREEZER RESCUE

We all have the best of intentions when we pack away those little containers of leftover foods and store them in the refrigerator. But often these receptacles are forgotten and the telltale aroma of something well past its prime soon makes its presence known, just a bit too late. Odors due to "expired" foods, or even up-to-date pungent smelling foods (like some cheeses) can create an offensive odor noticeable whenever the refrigerator door is opened. Strong odors can also affect fresh foods in both the refrigerator and the freezer.

If an unfriendly fragrance has permeated your freezer, remove all the contents and put them on ice in a cooler temporarily. If you have a separate temperature control for the freezer, turn it down for a few minutes. (If there isn't a separate control, leave the freezer door open for 5 minutes.) Wipe the interior of the freezer with a soft cloth dampened with a solution of ½ cup water, 3 tablespoons baking soda, and 6 drops eucalyptus or peppermint essential oil. Rinse well to remove any baking soda residue, and dry the walls, shelves, and floor of the freezer thoroughly with a tea towel before replacing food. Don't forget to turn the temperature control setting back up!

For refrigerator odors, you can use the solution recommended above to wipe down the walls, shelves, and doors, but increase the amount of essential oil to 10 drops.

Maintaining Freshness

If you just want to maintain freshness in the refrigerator, try one of these ideas:

■ Pour 2 ounces of vanilla extract (imitation is okay) into a small, shallow bowl or saucer and place it on a lower shelf for a few days.

■ If you like the smell of coffee, place a bowl of ½ cup ground coffee on a shelf. This will last for several weeks. You can add 5 to 7 drops of essential oil or even ground herbs, such as vanilla bean, sarsaparilla, mace, or ginger.

If you have a persistent odor in the refrigerator, try one of these tips:

■ Line the bottom shelf with newspaper that has been sprinkled with 10 to 15 drops of essential oil, such as lemon, lime, grapefruit, or sweet orange. Remove after 2 or 3 days.

- If you have an herb garden currently in bloom, cut a few stems of fragrant plants such as sage, rosemary, lemon balm, or mint. These can be tied with string and hung on an interior wall from one of those small plastic hooks with press-on backings available in any hardware store. The fresh herbs should last for 2 to 3 weeks.

- A slice of bread left on a plate will absorb many odors. You can sprinkle the bread slice with 2 to 4 drops of essential oil of your choice for extra deodorizing power.

KEEP THOSE CABINETS SPARKLING

If you have Formica cabinets in your kitchen, you can clean them with an all-purpose cleaner such as the formulas suggested in Cleaning Kitchen Appliances (page 49). The kitchen cabinets in our home are made of oak; for these I use a mixture of 2 cups water, ¼ cup Murphy's Oil Soap, and 15 to 20 drops of cedar or patchouli essential oil. The scent is heavenly — clean and "woodlike."

THE KITCHEN FLOOR

My sympathy goes to you if you chose or inherited light-colored flooring in your kitchen. With three boys, two cats, and a dog in our house, the kitchen traffic is nonstop and our old white flooring didn't keep any secrets about where they'd been. Thankfully, we now have multicolored patterned flooring in the kitchen that hardly shows a thing. Still, regardless of what kind of flooring there is in your kitchen it needs frequent washing, especially if there are human "floor dwellers" in your home. You can rest assured knowing that in addition to keeping your floor looking its best, these formulas are safe for young children who frequently crawl on them.

PINE-FRESH FLOOR CLEANER

This formula isn't at all like the old pine solvent cleaners you may be used to. It works just as well, but leaves a light scent more reminiscent of a pine forest than a bucket of chemicals. You can adjust the scent to your preference by increasing or reducing the amount of essential oil used.

- 1 gallon hot water
- 2 tablespoons liquid castile soap
- 10 drops pine essential oil
- 5 drops cypress essential oil

Combine all ingredients in a large bucket. Dip a mop into the bucket and squeeze out excess liquid. Clean the floor by working in sections, using short strokes and dipping the mop as needed. Rinsing is not necessary.

GET RID OF SCUFF MARKS

To remove scuff marks, apply 2 to 4 drops essential oil "neat" (undiluted) and wipe clean with a cloth. Rinse with a dash of vinegar.

Citrus Floor Cleaner

Nothing works like citrus in the kitchen!

> 1 gallon hot water
> 2 tablespoons liquid castile soap
> 15 drops sweet orange essential oil
> 8 drops lemon essential oil or ¼ cup lemon juice

Combine ingredients in a large bucket. Dip mop into the bucket and squeeze out excess liquid. Clean floor by working in sections, using short strokes and dipping mop as needed. Rinsing is not necessary.

Tough Dirt & Grease Formula

Put the grease-cutting power of vinegar to use with this excellent formula.

> 1 gallon hot water
> 2 tablespoons liquid castile soap
> ¼ cup washing soda
> 1 cup vinegar
> 20 drops eucalyptus, peppermint, or tea tree essential oil

Combine ingredients in a large bucket. Dip mop into the bucket and squeeze out excess liquid. Clean floor by working in sections, using short strokes and dipping mop as needed. Rinsing is not necessary.

HELPFUL HINTS FOR THE KITCHEN

Wipe up food spills in the oven as soon as possible. Better yet, line your oven with aluminum foil to prevent spills from caking on in the first place. Enamel stove tops can sometimes get those hard-to-wipe-off type of stains that only get worse as time goes on. But if you sprinkle on a few drops of your favorite essential oil the stain will wipe clean.

● ● ● ● ●

Sprinkle fresh grease spills in the oven with salt. When the oven has cooled, wipe clean with a soft cloth. Baking soda will also soak up the grease when applied this way.

● ● ● ● ●

Sanitize wooden cutting boards by rubbing with half of a freshly cut lemon, lime, or grapefruit. Or let the board soak in a solution of 2 cups of water and 15 drops of a citrus essential oil. Then wash with a mild soap and hot water.

● ● ● ● ●

Electric can openers can collect a lot of "gunk." Who wants to open a can of tuna for lunch after opening Fluffy and Fido's dinner the night before? Use an old, soft toothbrush dampened with 2 or 3 drops of any essential oil to clean in and between those small parts. Rinse, and the gunk is gone.

● ● ● ● ●

Keep garbage disposals smelling fresh by tossing in lemon, grapefruit, or lime remains when available.

● ● ● ● ●

How about some ready-when-you-need-'em kitchen wipes? Instead of using paper towels so frequently to wipe up spills or to clean off countertops, you can store multiple squares of soft cotton cloth or cellulose sponge in a container filled with a mixture of 1 cup water, 1 ounce liquid castile soap, and 6 to 8 drops of your favorite essential oil. The cloths, made from old T-shirts or pajamas, can be washed and returned to the jar for reuse. Be sure to cap the jar between uses.

* * * * *

Keep a supply of 100 percent cotton cloths and towels on hand to use instead of paper towels.

To reduce your consumption of paper napkins, use cloth napkins and placemats whenever possible.

* * * * *

Plastic storage containers can get heavily stained from foods such as tomato sauce, especially if they're frequently microwaved to reheat leftovers. For these stains, let the containers soak in a strong herbal infusion (I use lemon balm, mint, or sage, which grow profusely in our garden) and a tablespoon of baking soda. After soaking for an hour or so, scrub the container with a little more baking soda if needed. The stains may not disappear entirely, but they're bound to look better than before.

* * * * *

Reduce your use of plastic wrap, aluminum foil, and brown paper bags by using plastic containers to tote lunches to work or school. That goes for plastic tableware as well. All are dishwasher safe; with proper care they can last for years. And plastic containers can always be used to store other materials when they are "retired" from kitchen service.

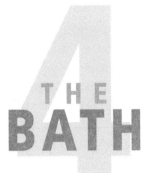

THE BATH 4

Due to the nature of things we do there, the bathroom is a breeding ground for germs. Other than the obvious activities, there's also a lot of hair brushing, sloughing of dry skin, and other body-care rituals with the potential for mold and mildew making. If you have more than one bathroom, there's more of the same going on there. These formulas are gentle on your hands and get the job done without harmful chemicals.

MOLD & MILDEW BUSTERS

Mold and mildew are always a threat, especially if there is a window with a sill in your bathroom. The steam from showers and baths can affect the woodwork of the window and lead to peeling paint and mildew spots. Ventilation, such as an exhaust fan, can help minimize this problem.

The same applies to the shower curtain. The best kind of shower curtain to buy is a cloth type that can be laundered. Hang it to dry in the sun to thwart mildew and bacteria.

HERBAL DISINFECTANT

A super disinfectant formula that's incredibly easy to make.

> 2 cups hot water
> 5 sprigs fresh thyme or 10 drops thyme essential oil
> ¼ cup borax

If using the fresh herb, bring the water to a boil and pour over the thyme sprigs in a bowl. Allow to steep for 30 minutes and then strain off liquid into a spray bottle. Add borax and shake well. If using the essential oil, combine all ingredients in a spray bottle and shake well. Spray on surfaces and wipe clean with a damp cloth or sponge.

PINE DISINFECTANT

You'll definitely prefer this recipe to your old "pine" cleaner.

> 2 cups water
> 2 teaspoons borax
> 8 drops pine essential oil
> 4 drops cedar essential oil

Combine all ingredients in a clean spray bottle. Shake before each use. Spray onto bathroom surfaces and wipe clean with a damp cloth or sponge.

MOLD & MILDEW PREVENTION FORMULA

Use this formula on shower stalls and curtains, the tracks between sliding glass doors, and other moist areas.

> 2 cups water
> 8–10 drops citrus seed extract
> 2 teaspoons tea tree essential oil
> 4 drops juniper essential oil

Combine all ingredients in a spray bottle. Spray areas and surfaces well but do not rinse. *Note:* If you already have a buildup of mold or mildew, allow the spray to "rest" on the surface areas for a few hours. Wipe with a soft cloth, then respray the areas and let dry without rinsing.

MOLD DETERRENT

If you already have a buildup of mold or mildew, allow the spray to "rest" on the surface areas for a few hours. Wipe with a soft cloth, then respray the areas and let dry without rinsing.

> 1¼ cups white vinegar
> ¾ cup water
> 4 drops cinnamon essential oil
> 6 drops patchouli essential oil
> 2 teaspoons tea tree essential oil

Combine all ingredients in a spray bottle. Spray surfaces well but do not rinse.

SCOURING POWDERS & CLEANSERS

The following cleaners possess sanitizing and antibacterial qualities while offering a variety of herbal scents. You can make larger batches of these products and store them in plastic containers. (Large plastic spice jars with shaker tops work great for this purpose.)

Herbal Scouring Powder for Sinks

This powder rubs out grime while leaving a fresh, earthy scent. Make sure you rinse well to remove any residue.

> 1 cup baking soda
> ¼ cup dried sage leaves, ground
> ¼ cup rosemary leaves, crushed
> 1 teaspoon cream of tartar

Combine all ingredients in a plastic container, preferably one with a shaker top. Shake well. Sprinkle a small amount of the powder into sink and scrub with a damp sponge or cloth. Rinse well with plain water.

Whitening Scouring Powder

The combination of borax and citrus peel will kill germs and remove stains.

> 1 cup baking soda
> 2 teaspoons cream of tartar
> ⅛ cup borax
> ¼ cup grated lemon, orange, or
>   grapefruit peel

Combine all ingredients in a plastic container, preferably one with a shaker top. Shake well. Sprinkle a small amount of the powder into sink and scrub with a damp sponge or cloth. Rinse well with plain water.

FRAGRANT SCOURING POWDER

This formula has a clean, pleasant scent. Increase the amount of rosemary essential oil to 4 drops for more fragrance.

> 1 cup baking soda
> ¼ cup rose petals, crushed
> 2 drops rosemary essential oil

Combine all ingredients in a plastic container, preferably one with a shaker top. Shake well. Sprinkle a small amount of the powder into sink and scrub with a damp sponge or cloth. Rinse well.

LEMONY SCOURING POWDER

This is the formula for lemon lovers! And with this combination of herbs, germs don't stand a chance.

> 1 cup baking soda
> ¼ cup crushed, dried lemon balm leaves
> 3 drops lemon or lemongrass essential oil
> 3 drops citronella essential oil or grapefruit seed extract

Combine all ingredients in a container, preferably one with a shaker top. Shake well. Sprinkle powder onto surface and scrub with a damp cloth or sponge. Rinse well.

EARTHY SCOURING POWDER

This cleanser will make you think you're tending your garden instead of cleaning the bathroom. The dried rosemary leaves lend extra scrubbing action.

> 1 cup baking soda
> ¼ cup dried, crushed rosemary leaves
> 5 drops thyme essential oil
> 3 drops oregano essential oil

Combine all ingredients in a container, preferably one with a shaker top. Shake well. Sprinkle powder onto surface and scrub with a damp cloth or sponge. Rinse well.

Tub & Tile Soft Scrubber

A used plastic dishwashing liquid or shampoo bottle with a squirt top is an ideal container for your scrubber.

- 1 cup baking soda
- ¼ cup liquid castile soap
- 2 vitamin C tablets, crushed
- 3-5 drops eucalyptus or tea tree essential oil
- water

Combine baking soda, soap, vitamin C, and essential oil in a plastic bottle. Add just enough water to make a smooth liquid paste. Shake or stir to mix. Apply paste to surface and rub with a damp cloth or sponge until area is clean. Rinse several times with water.

Lavender Soft Scrubber

This scrubber not only cleans, but is mild and will actually soften your hands!

- ¾ cup baking soda
- ¼ cup powdered milk
- ⅛ cup liquid castile soap
- 5 drops lavender essential oil
- water

Combine baking soda, milk, castile soap, and lavender oil in a squirt-top bottle. Add just enough water to make a smooth paste. Shake or stir to mix. Apply to surface, then wipe area clean with a damp sponge or cloth. Rinse well.

FIZZY BATHROOM SINK CLEANER

Kids love to watch the "volcanic" action that occurs after pouring the vinegar over the baking soda. Who knows? You might even get your kids to clean the bathroom!

> ½ cup baking soda
> 6 drops lemon or lime essential oil
> ¼ cup vinegar

Combine the baking soda and essential oil. Sprinkle into the sink; pour the vinegar on top. After the fizz settles, scrub clean with a damp cloth or sponge. Rinse clean.

SOAP SCUM REMOVER

This is a formula to remove that annoying buildup that forms on soap dishes and toothbrush holders. The vinegar will produce a "fizzing" action.

> 1 tablespoon baking soda
> 1 teaspoon salt
> 2 drops essential oil of choice
> vinegar

Combine baking soda, salt, and essential oil in a small cup. Add just enough vinegar to make a paste. Apply to surface and scrub with a damp cloth or sponge. Rinse well.

SANITIZING THE TOILET

One of the most important areas in the bathroom to clean, of course, is the commode. Most people think that the bowl itself is where the real "nasties" hide, but actually, it's relatively clean. Most germs take refuge behind and under the seat. Since this is the part being handled most often, it needs careful and frequent sanitizing. There are some excellent bacteria busters offered here to do just that.

Germs-Be-Gone Toilet Cleaner

This is an antibacterial spray cleaner especially formulated for cleaning the general surface area of the toilet and under and behind the seat.

> 2 cups water
> ¼ cup liquid castile soap
> 1 tablespoon tea tree essential oil
> 10 drops eucalyptus or peppermint essential oil

Combine all ingredients in a plastic spray bottle and shake well. Spray on toilet surfaces and wipe clean with a damp cloth or sponge.

No-Scrub Toilet Bowl Cleaner

This is for toilet bowls that have an everlasting ring around them. (Like the kind you find in the bathroom of your vacation cabin after six months of nonuse.) You can employ this recipe just before going to bed; by morning, even the toughest of stains will have disappeared.

> 1 cup borax
> 1 cup vinegar
> 10 drops pine or lavender essential oil
> 5 drops lemon or lime essential oil

Combine all ingredients in a plastic bowl or bottle and pour all at once into the toilet bowl. Allow to sit overnight. In the morning, just flush!

EASY-DOES-IT BOWL CLEANER

What could be simpler than this easy and effective formula?

> ½ cup baking soda
> ¼ cup white vinegar
> 10 drops tea tree essential oil

Combine all ingredients. Just add to the bowl, swipe with a brush, and you're done.

MIRROR BRIGHT

This mixture not only cleans the mirror (and faucets) to a shine, but it will help to prevent fogging while the shower is running.

> 1½ cups vinegar
> ½ cup water
> 8 drops citrus essential oil of choice

Combine all ingredients in a spray bottle and shake well before use. Spray solution onto mirror and wipe with a dry cloth or towel.

HELPFUL HINTS FOR THE BATHROOM

To maintain a fresh scent in the bathroom, place a few drops of your favorite essential oil on the cardboard tube supporting the toilet paper. Every time the paper is used, the fragrance will be released.

● ● ● ● ●

Place a bowl of potpourri on the sink or toilet tank. Replace the potpourri every three months. For recipes, see chapter 9. Potpourri, whether made from natural or synthetic materials, can be toxic to pets and young children who might be tempted to handle or even eat it. If this scenario is a possibility in your home, you can place the potpourri on a high shelf. Or try filling a muslin or cloth bag with the potpourri, then hang it out of reach.

* * * * *

To keep bath mats and rugs smelling fresh between washings, simply scent ½ cup baking soda with 8 to 10 drops of the essential oil of your choice. Sprinkle on the carpets, wait 15 minutes, and then vacuum.

* * * * *

If you have a stand-alone toothbrush holder, be sure to run it through the dishwasher often. You'd be amazed at the germs and dirt that thrive there. If it's really full of gunk, let it stand for 20 minutes filled with water and two or three drops of tea tree essential oil. Then wash by hand or in the dishwasher.

* * * * *

Don't forget to periodically clean combs and hairbrushes. Let them stand for 20 minutes in a container with 1½ cups water, ½ cup vinegar, and 20 drops of tea tree, rosemary, lavender, or eucalyptus essential oil. Rinse well and allow to air-dry before putting them away.

THE
LAUNDRY

Manufacturers of laundry products spend a good deal of money on advertising to convince us that their products contain "magical" ingredients that can solve every laundry problem. Well, they don't. With their cleaning power stemming from caustic bleach, EDTA, and optical brighteners (which are strong allergens), their ingredients are anything but magical. But the fact is, many commercial laundry soaps contain nearly 70 percent ordinary washing soda. The difference between them basically comes down to fragrance, color, and variations in the amount of additives.

SIMPLE LAUNDRY GUIDELINES

Before you can properly clean your dirty laundry, you need to consider what you want your washer and detergent to accomplish. It doesn't do any good to wash heavily soiled work clothes with the baby's pajamas, as oils can transfer from one to the other. Likewise, you can't expect your white shirt to easily free itself of a coffee stain if you're going to wait three days before washing it. So before you even lift the lid of the washer, there are some basic laundry guidelines to follow to help preserve your garments and keep them looking their best.

Sorting Laundry

Your mother probably told you never to wash colored clothes with white ones. But she might not have told you that there's a lot more to sorting laundry. Here are some considerations when sorting:

- The first step is to sort by color. Whites, very bright colors (such as red or orange), pastels, and dark colors should be washed separately. Next, sort heavy fabrics from delicate garments that must be laundered in the gentle cycle.
- Towels, sheets, and bedspreads should be washed separately because they produce lint that will adhere to other fabrics, such as knits.
- Don't forget to check the pockets of your children's jeans, jackets, and shirts! I've been surprised many times by the array of trinkets a child can collect in his pockets, including coins and partially eaten foodstuffs. On one memorable

occasion, a broken ballpoint pen remained undetected until it had been through the dryer! (Although the inside of the dryer ended up with a polka-dot pattern, the ink wiped away easily with a rag moistened with vinegar and cedar essential oil.)

Before You Wash

Pretreating is all-important if you really want to rid your clothes of stains and heavy soiling. These are the best stain-fighting tactics:

■ Pretreat stains as soon as possible; this is the golden rule of the laundry room. Always rinse a stain in cold water — warm water can cause fruit and sugar stains to set in. See pages 78–79 for pretreatment formulas.

■ Prewash heavily soiled items to help eliminate most of the dirt without redepositing it on clothes. After running clothes through the prewash cycle, drain and wash in the regular cycle — in hot water if the fabric permits it.

■ Presoak old or tough stains like blood and grass for 30 minutes or more.

Water Temperature

Your washing machine comes equipped with a water temperature control for a reason: not all fabrics are created equal. Always follow specific instructions given on a garment's care label. To avoid damaging garments, remember:

■ Washing in cold water will prevent shrinking and the release of dyes. Bright colors, lightly soiled items, and delicate garments should be washed in cold water. Rinsing in cold water is suitable for all types of laundry. And you'll be saving energy, too.

■ Warm water helps to reduce wrinkling and the bleeding of colors. Choose warm water washing for permanent press, washable wool, dark colors, and synthetic fabrics.

■ Hot water is recommended for heavily soiled clothing, towels, whites, pastels, and light-colored prints. Never wash 100 percent cotton or 100 percent wool items in hot water or they will shrink. Instead, use cold water for cotton and hand wash wool items.

The Detergent Dilemma

Believe it or not, you're probably using more laundry product than you need per load. How much do you really need to use? The usual recommended capful is almost twice as much as you need for an average load. In fact, excess detergent leads to residue that only traps dirt in the clothes you've just washed. It's not only environmentally friendly to use less, it's easier on your clothing and your budget too.

Here are some other detergent tips:

■ Keep a big jug of white vinegar in your laundry area. It makes blankets soft and fluffy and dissolves uric acid, making it perfect for washing babies' items. Vinegar also reduces soap residue, breaks up grease and oil, and is a natural bleach. As an added benefit, washing clothes in vinegar can help prevent static cling in the dryer.

- Laundry soap doesn't perform as well in hard water, but this can be corrected by adding zeolite powder, orrisroot, baking soda, or borax to the wash.

- If you can locate soap flakes, buy them in bulk! Soap flakes are hard to find in supermarkets, and Ivory Snow is no longer pure soap flakes; it became a detergent in 1991. If you can't find packages of soap flakes, you can grate your own flakes from bars of soap. Bars of pure castile soap can be found in most natural foods stores and some supermarkets.

THE HERBAL TOUCH

Herbal essential oils can be blended into laundry formulas (liquid or powder) or added to the softener dispenser of your machine. Essential oils not only boost cleaning power, they also provide a fresh, clean scent.

Essential oils can also lend therapeutic qualities. For instance, add tea tree essential oil to your laundry if you suffer from frequent yeast infections. Eucalyptus essential oil can be used when someone in the household is fighting a cold. Jasmine, rose, or ylang-ylang essential oil will impart a romantic scent to fine washables. You are encouraged to experiment! You can even create your own unique blend from the essential oil chart on the following page.

Herbal-scented baking soda is another way to use essential oils in the laundry. Baking soda adds whitening power and is a natural water softener.

For a 16-ounce box, use 15 to 20 drops of essential oil. You can mix it right in the box! Simply add the oils to the box and shake well. Or add 3 to 5 drops of essential oil to 1 cup of white vinegar; the oil lends additional cleaning power and helps to remove odors.

Be creative in your thinking, and you'll soon find that you don't miss store-bought detergents at all.

ESSENTIAL OIL CHART
FOR LAUNDRY

All of these essential oils help clean and freshen the laundry. They offer other benefits as well.

Essential Oil	Benefit
Cedar	Adds a clean, woodsy scent
Chamomile	Soothing
Eucalyptus	Excellent for colds and sinus trouble
Lavender	Relaxing
Lemon	Stimulating, helps whiten laundry
Peppermint	Good for colds and sinus trouble
Rose geranium	Adds a romatic scent
Rosemary*	Calming (but often stimulating on its own)
Sweet orange	Helps remove stains and whiten laundry
Tea tree	Antibacterial and antifungal

*Not suitable for wool, silk, or satin

MAKING NATURAL LAUNDRY SOAPS

These formulas don't have any magical components that you can't pronounce. Instead, the cleaning power of these soaps comes from combining clean, pure ingredients.

BASIC LAUNDRY SOAP POWDER

This recipe will wash six average loads, but you can easily double it.

> 1 cup washing soda
> 1 cup scented baking soda (see essential oil chart for selection)
> 1 cup soap flakes or *finely* grated pure bar soap

Blend all ingredients and store in a heavy plastic container. Use ½ cup for an average laundry load.

BASIC LAUNDRY SOAP LIQUID

The addition of glycerin and essential oil gives extra cleaning power while still being gentle on clothing.

> 1 ounce liquid castile soap
> 2 tablespoons glycerin
> 1 cup washing soda
> 1 cup baking soda
> 2 cups warm water
> 10 drops essential oil of choice

Combine all ingredients in a heavy plastic container (don't use plastic milk containers — they're not heavy enough) and shake well before using. Use ¼ to ½ cup, depending on the size of the load and how dirty the clothes are.

HARD WATER FORMULA

Hard water can affect the performance of your laundry soap. This formula uses borax and vinegar as natural water softeners.

> 1 cup soap flakes or *finely* grated pure bar soap
> 1 cup washing soda
> ½ cup borax
> 2 cups vinegar
> 10 drops essential oil of choice

Combine the soap, washing soda, and borax in a heavy plastic container. Blend the vinegar and essential oils in a separate container, preferably one with a pour spout. Use ½ cup of the soap mixture for washing; add ½ cup of the vinegar mixture during the rinse cycle.

FINE WASHABLES FORMULA

Rosemary is an old favorite for freshening delicate knits and lingerie. Note: Do not use on items that are 100 percent wool, silk, or satin.

> 1 ounce liquid castile soap
> 1 cup rosemary infusion

The rosemary infusion can be made a few different ways. If you have fresh rosemary, you can steep two sprigs of "bruised" rosemary (slightly crushed between the fingers to release the oils) in 1 cup of boiling water for 15 minutes, then strain. Or steep 1 teaspoon of dried, crushed rosemary leaves in 1 cup boiling water for 15 minutes, then strain. If using essential oil, add 3 drops to 1 cup of hot water. Place the clothes in the washer and add the castile soap and rosemary infusion. Launder in cold water on the gentle cycle.

DIAPER WHITENER

Add ½ cup borax, ¼ cup vinegar, and 6 to 8 drops of essential oil to a pail or bucket of hot water. Soak diapers for 20 to 30 minutes, or more if heavily soiled, before laundering.

BABY'S LAUNDRY FORMULA

Babies can sure get their clothing messy! Borax and vinegar will help to whiten and soften fabrics.

>   2 drops essential oil (optional)
>   2 tablespoons liquid castile soap
>   ¼ cup washing soda
>   1 cup baking soda
>   ¼ cup borax

If using essential oil, mix with the castile soap. Add this mixture to washer along with the washing soda, baking soda, and borax. Launder as usual.

BRIGHT COLORS FORMULA

This recipe makes enough for one load. You can make larger batches, but keep the liquid castile soap separate.

>   1 ounce liquid castile soap (scented with
>   2 to 4 drops essential oil, if desired)
>   ¼ cup washing soda
>   ½ cup Epsom salts

Add the liquid castile soap to washer, then add washing soda and Epsom salts. Launder as usual.

BLEACH ALTERNATIVE FORMULA

This formula makes enough for one load of laundry. You can make larger batches, but keep the lemon juice mixture separate until ready to use.

> ½ cup Basic Laundry Soap Liquid (page 74)
> ¼ cup borax
> ¼ cup lemon juice or vinegar, plus 6 drops lemon essential oil

Combine all ingredients in a heavy plastic jug or other container of choice. For extra whitening power, let the clean clothes hang outside to dry in the sun.

Natural Fabrics Rescue

Natural fabrics, such as wool and silk, need special care. Wool should be hand washed in cool water and a capful of liquid castile soap, then rinsed well in a tub of clean water. Never allow wool to soak. Nor should you attempt to wring wool dry. After the final rinse, place the wool garment on a dry towel and roll up like a jelly roll. Gently press on the towel to remove excess water. Repeat this process if necessary with another towel. Then place the garment flat on a dry towel, reshape, and leave it to dry.

Silk items should be dipped in a solution of warm water and a capful of liquid castile soap. Rinse well and gently squeeze out excess water. Turn the garment inside out and hang until it is just damp to the touch. With the garment still reversed, press with an iron on low setting.

PRETREATMENTS FOR STAINS

Since vinegar can remove some dyes, test these formulas on a small area of the fabric before treating the actual stain.

PERSPIRATION STAIN REMOVER

Use this formula to pretreat ring around the collar and perspiration stains.

> ¼ cup vinegar
> 4 drops lemon, lime, or eucalyptus
>   essential oil
> 1 tablespoon baking soda

Combine all ingredients. Rub the mixture into the stains with your fingers, a soft cloth, or an old toothbrush. Launder as usual.

PERSPIRATION PRESOAK #1

Try this fresh-smelling pretreatment before you wash.

> 1 cup vinegar
> ¼ cup lemon juice
> 6 drops tea tree essential oil

Combine all ingredients and add to the clothes in a washer full of warm water. Allow to soak for an hour or two, then wash as usual.

PERSPIRATION PRESOAK #2

This is another great vinegar-based stain remover.

> 1 cup vinegar
> ½ cup salt
> 3 drops tea tree essential oil

Place clothes in washer and add enough warm water to cover them. Combine all ingredients and add to washer. Let clothes soak for an hour or more, then wash as usual.

All-Purpose Stain Spray

Since food and drink spills aren't likely to occur while you're in the laundry room, why not make up extra bottles and keep this formula handy in the kitchen and bath as well?

- ¼ cup vegetable oil–based soap
- ¼ cup glycerin
- 2 tablespoons borax
- 10 drops peppermint or tea tree essential oil
- 1¾ cups water

Combine all ingredients in a spray bottle and shake well. Spray generously onto stain. Launder as usual.

On-the-Spot Stain Lifter

Accidents happen, but this stain remover will make you forget the stain was ever there.

- 2 tablespoons cream of tartar
- 2 drops peppermint, eucalyptus, or lemon essential oil
- water

Combine all ingredients in a small cup, using just enough water to make a paste. Spread the paste over the stain and allow it to dry completely before washing.

FABRIC SOFTENERS

Vinegar is the fabric softener of choice for many reasons. Not only is it nontoxic, it also removes soap residue in the rinse cycle and helps to prevent static cling in the dryer. The fun part is in using different scented vinegars. Essential oils can produce a fresh, clean, floral, woodsy, or spicy effect — use whatever fragrance suits your fancy.

Adding one or two cups of vinegar to the rinse cycle is fine for whites, but more than that can cause some dyes to run, especially from rayon fabrics. Keep the color and fabric in mind when using these formulas.

LAVENDER FABRIC SOFTENER

Formulas don't get much easier than this one, which is both fragrant and effective.

> 1 gallon vinegar
> 20 drops lavender essential oil

Add the lavender essential oil to the vinegar right in the container and you've got instant fabric softener! Shake well before using. For a large load, add 1 cup during the rinse cycle; use ½ cup during the rinse cycle for smaller loads.

MINTY-FRESH FABRIC SOFTENER

This formula helps remove tough odors from clothing.

> 1 gallon vinegar
> 10 drops peppermint essential oil

Combine ingredients in a heavy-duty plastic container. Add 1 cup to the rinse cycle for each load.

LEMONY FABRIC SOFTENER

There's nothing like the smell of lemons to suggest freshness.

> 6 cups vinegar
> 1 cup water
> 1 cup baking soda
> 15 drops lemon or lemongrass essential oil

Combine all ingredients in a heavy-duty plastic container. Add 1 cup to the rinse cycle for each load for truly lemon-fresh clothes.

DRYER SHEETS

This is a clever and simple idea — natural dryer sheets can be made from a scrap of cotton cloth and 3 to 5 drops of your favorite essential oil. Using more may actually soil your newly washed laundry. Here are some interesting combinations you could try:

- Cedar and patchouli for a masculine, woodsy scent
- Rosemary and thyme for an earthy scent
- Geranium and neroli (orange blossom) for a floral scent
- Peppermint and eucalyptus for cold sufferers
- Jasmine and ylang ylang for a romantic scent
- Sweet orange and lemon for a refreshing scent
- Chamomile and hyssop for a relaxing effect (helps insomnia!)

To a scrap of cotton cloth (about 4 inches square), add 3 to 5 drops of your favorite essential oil. Toss into the dryer with the rest of the laundry. You can use the same cloth two or three times, each time refreshing it with 3 more drops essential oil. After that, wash the cloth and it's ready to be used again.

LAUNDRY STARCH

Here's a quick alternative to the commercial, chemical-laden starches.

> 1 cup water
> 2 tablespoons cornstarch
> 2 drops essential oil of choice (use a clear oil like tea tree for light colors)
> ½ cup cooled black tea (for darker colors *only*)

Combine all ingredients in a spray bottle. Shake well before each use. Lightly spray garment and iron as usual.

LAUNDRY PROBLEM-SOLVERS

Sometimes, real life happens and we can't always tend to a stain right away. Or the stain is the worst you can ask for, such as red wine, blood, or ink. But before you toss the garment out or make it into a dusting cloth, give one of these natural remedies a try. If a stain doesn't come out the first time, it's worth repeating the process. Whatever you do, don't put the garment into the dryer if the stain is still visible after air-drying; doing so could make the stain permanent.

The following is a list of the most troublesome types of stains and some suggested remedies. Some of these stain problem-solvers involve herbal teas or extracts, while some call for other easy-to-use natural ingredients that you probably have on hand.

Baby formula. Anyone who has cared for an infant knows that formula, especially those that are soy-based, makes an ugly stain. But if formula stains are treated when they land on clothing, they can sometimes leave a ring after laundering. To treat them, rub a mixture of vinegar and a few drops of garlic juice into the stain. This will help to break down the protein in the formula and release it from the fabric. A little moistened meat tenderizer will do the same thing. I also discovered long ago that baby wipes — which are basically a combination of alcohol, mild cleanser, and emollients — will remove these stains beautifully if applied right away, and are safe for most fabrics. Choose the method best for the age of the stain and the type of fabric that you're treating.

◦ ◦ ● ◦ ◦

Berries. If the stain is fresh, rub a slice of lemon over it several times. If the stain is old, treat it with glycerin and wait 30 minutes. Rinse and allow to air-dry. If the stain endures, make a mixture of 1 heaping tablespoon cornstarch, 2 drops eucalyptus essential oil, and 1 teaspoon glycerin. Add just enough water to make a thick paste and spread on the stain. Without rinsing, put the garment in the sun to dry. Repeat the paste application if necessary. Once the stain is gone you can launder as usual.

◦ ◦ ● ◦ ◦

Blood. Immediately rinse the garment thoroughly in cool water. If necessary, let the garment soak in a solution of laundry soap and water for several hours. For light-colored fabrics, try wiping with a soft cloth moistened with hydrogen peroxide. Hang the garment in the sun and keep applying hydrogen peroxide until all traces of the stain are gone. Allow to dry and launder as usual.

* * * * *

Butter or margarine. Make a paste of 1 tablespoon baking soda, 2 drops lemon, lime, or orange essential oil, and water. Spread the paste on the stain and allow to dry, then wash as usual.

* * * * *

Candle wax. First harden the wax with ice cubes and gently peel off as much as you can. Then place the stained area between paper towels and press with a warm iron. Keep moving or replacing the paper towels to avoid transferring the candle wax back into the fabric. Continue this procedure until the paper towels no longer absorb the wax. The remaining stain should then be treated with a little glycerin on a cotton ball and laundered as usual.

* * * * *

Chewing gum. If chewing gum makes its way onto clothing, put the garment in a plastic bag and place in the freezer for 30 to 45 minutes. The gum should pull right off. If a residue remains, soak in full-strength vinegar before washing.

* * * * *

Chocolate. Make a paste of borax and water and spread over the stain. Allow to dry and then launder as usual.

Coffee and tea. Immediately flush with cool water. Then soak in a borax and water solution before laundering.

· · · · ·

Egg. Scrape off any dried material. Douse the remaining stain with a mixture of 2 teaspoons lemon juice and 3 drops sweet orange or lemon essential oil. Wash in cold water.

· · · · ·

Grass. Soak garment in vinegar, then spread a paste of baking soda and water over the stain. Wash in hot water.

· · · · ·

Grease. Cover the stain with a mixture of 2 teaspoons each of cornmeal, salt, and baking soda. Let this mixture stand for 30 minutes or more to absorb as much grease as possible, then wipe away. Soak the remaining stain in ½ cup vinegar, 5 drops lemon or orange essential oil or grapefruit seed extract, and ¼ cup water until the stain breaks free. If the fabric can tolerate it, wash in hot water.

· · · · ·

Ink. Place a cloth under the fabric and dab the stain repeatedly with undiluted eucalyptus essential oil until it begins to break up. The ink will begin to transfer to the underlying cloth. Remove as much of the stain as you can with this method. Then soak the garment in a solution of equal parts of vinegar and milk before washing.

Linens. Linens can sometimes yellow if stored in a trunk or closet for a long time. The best prevention is to wrap them carefully in acid-free paper before storing. If yellowing does occur you can soak them in a tea made from 2 or 3 fresh rhubarb stalks and 3 cups boiling water. Allow the material to dry in the sun. Repeat as necessary until the stains have disappeared. You can also use 1 cup lemon juice diluted in 2 cups water in place of the rhubarb tea.

• • • • •

Lipstick. Gently massage the stain with white toothpaste or 3 to 4 drops of glycerin for a few minutes and blot dry. Then wipe several times with eucalyptus essential oil. Launder as usual. Repeat the eucalyptus application if the stain doesn't come out completely after washing.

• • • • •

Mold and mildew. Sometimes towels are left in a duffel bag after a day at the beach, or clothes are put into storage while still damp, resulting in mold or mildew stains. Pretreat these stains with a solution of ¼ cup vinegar, 1 teaspoon salt, and 6 drops tea tree essential oil. Launder as usual.

• • • • •

Mustard. Mustard contains turmeric, which yields a bright yellow dye. To break up the stain, apply some glycerin and let stand for 30 minutes. Then gently massage some laundry soap (liquid or powder) into the stain and wash as usual.

Nail polish. First try blotting the stain with rubbing alcohol. If this doesn't work, test some nail polish remover in an inconspicuous place on the garment. If the test area of the fabric isn't damaged, proceed to the stain. *Note:* Organic nail polish removers are available at health food stores that carry natural cosmetics.

* * * * *

Oil. Carefully blot up excess oil from the garment, then follow the treatment recommended for grease stains.

* * * * *

Paint. Success depends on the type of paint involved. Latex paint is easily removed by rinsing in hot soapy water. Oil-based paint is another matter, and your best chance is to act immediately. Rub the stain with rubbing alcohol, then soak in a solution of equal parts hot vinegar and milk for several hours. If this doesn't work, you may have to take the garment to a professional cleaner or accept the fact that it's now a dust cloth.

* * * * *

Pencil. Pencil marks may seem innocent, but they can persist after washing. The cure is simple: Rub them off with an eraser before washing.

* * * * *

Rust. One way to remove rust is to make a paste of lemon juice and salt. Let the paste sit on the stain for several minutes and then pour boiling water over the stain. Another method is to boil the garment in 1 tablespoon cream of tartar and 1 quart of water. An old-fashioned but time-tested remedy for rust stains is to let the fabric soak in a cooled "tea" made from 2 to 3 fresh rhubarb stalks and 3 cups boiling water.

* * * * *

Salad dressing. Soak in a solution of ½ cup vinegar, ½ cup lemon juice, and 6 to 8 drops of sweet orange, eucalyptus, or tea tree essential oil for 30 minutes. Then launder as usual, in hot water if the fabric permits it.

* * * * *

Scorch marks. For light-colored fabrics, test a small area with hydrogen peroxide. If no damage occurs, treat the stain by dabbing on hydrogen peroxide, then hang the garment in direct sunlight. Keep the stain moistened with additional hydrogen peroxide until the scorch marks fade. For darker clothing, coat the stain with glycerin and allow to "rest" overnight. Then wash as usual. If any residue from the glycerin remains after washing, it can be removed by rubbing with liquid castile soap and rinsing thoroughly.

* * * * *

Shoe polish. Water or any other "wet" treatment will cause this stain to spread. Instead, *blot* the stain with glycerin on a soft, clean cloth to loosen it from the garment's fibers, then launder as usual.

Tar. Fresh tar can be countered by first scraping off surface pieces with a warm butter knife. Dried tar should first be treated with glycerin or olive oil to soften it. Then place the garment over several folded paper towels and pour on 2 or 3 drops of eucalyptus essential oil. The paper towels will absorb the dissolving tar underneath, so replace them as needed. Keep working with the knife during this process to scrape off the lifting tar. Repeat this process until the tar has been removed.

* * * * *

Urine. Soak the material in a solution of 1 cup vinegar, 5 drops lavender essential oil, and, if the fabric can tolerate it, 1 cup very hot water for 30 minutes. Then wash as usual.

* * * * *

Wine. Rinse in cool water right away, then follow the procedure for removing berry stains.

WOOD CARE

IN THIS CHAPTER

Cleaners • Dusters • Polishes
Waxes • Helpful Hints

It isn't necessary to use an oily product every time you dust your furniture. In fact, some types of furniture never need oil, just a dusting with a damp cloth. It depends on the type of finish put on the furniture, if any at all.

Since most furniture made today has a finish that doesn't absorb oil, your objective is to remove dirt and dust, not to leave an oily surface for dust to thrive on. Some older pieces and unfinished wood, however, can benefit from an occasional oil treatment. Always test wood cleaning formulas on an inconspicuous area of your furniture, like the inside of a leg or a panel underneath, before treating the entire piece. This is a very important step, as some essential oils can adversely affect certain wood finishes.

It's the same story with hardwood flooring — some floors are given a surface finish and others a penetrating finish. If your hardwood floor has a shiny, glossy appearance, it probably has a coating of varnish, such as polyurethane. For this type of flooring, regular cleaning with a vegetable-oil wood soap will remove any surface dirt and restore a high sheen. If your floor doesn't come back to life after cleaning, it may need a new surface finish. If your floor has a slightly oily feel when you draw your hand across it, it likely has a penetrating finish and needs additional waxing now and then to protect it.

Approach wood paneling with caution; it can be damaged by the application of liquids. Most wood paneling only requires occasional dusting with a soft cloth. If it has an oily finish however, you can mist the cloth with a cleaner such as Cedarwood Dusting Aid (see page 93) or an oily cleaner such as Mositure-Rich Duster (see page 94). As with flooring or wood furniture, test the formula on a small area first.

WOOD CLEANERS

These formulas are for furniture with a hard finish and in need of a good surface cleaning, like garage and estate sale finds, or items kept in storage for a long time. If cleaning the wood doesn't revive the piece, it may be time for refinishing.

FRAGRANT WOOD CLEANER

This fragrant formula will clear away sticky grime. Using bergamot or geranium essential oil will give a floral scent.

> ½ cup lemon juice
> 1 teaspoon liquid castile soap
> 4 drops bergamot, geranium, or sweet orange essential oil

Combine all ingredients in a small spray bottle. Apply to wood and wipe clean with a damp cloth. Wipe again with a dry cloth.

BERRY GOOD FOR WOOD CLEANER

Use this fruity solution to bring dingy, dull wood furniture back to life.

> 1 tablespoon fresh raspberry leaves
> 1 cup boiling water
> ½ cup vinegar
> ½ cup lemon juice

Steep raspberry leaves in water for 20 minutes. Strain. In a spray bottle, combine tea, vinegar, and lemon juice. Shake well. Moisten a soft cloth with the solution and gently rub the wood to loosen and remove dirt. Use a second clean cloth dampened with water to remove any residue. Wipe again with a dry towel.

DUSTING AIDS

These formulas are useful for regular dusting, and they smell great too. Choose one that's right for the type of wood you have.

Lemon-Fresh Dust Buster

This recipe is for a single use. You could make larger quantities, but the presence of lemon juice necessitates refrigeration. If you want to make enough to store in a spray bottle, you could increase the amount of lemon balm tea to 2 cups, omit the lemon juice, and increase the lemon essential oil to 20 drops.

¼ cup lemon juice
⅛ cup cooled lemon balm tea
2 drops thyme essential oil
4 drops lemon essential oil

Combine all ingredients in a spray bottle and shake well. Spray onto wood and wipe clean with a dry cloth.

Cedarwood Dusting Aid

This is my personal favorite! I use it for bookcases, coffee tables, kitchen cabinets, and the antique dining room table that we refinished a few years back. I adore the scent of cedar on wood; the sweet orange oil adds just the right touch. This recipe makes enough for a large spray bottle.

½ cup oil soap (I like Murphy's Oil Soap)
¾ cup water
5 drops sweet orange or patchouli
  essential oil
15–20 drops cedar essential oil

Combine all ingredients in a spray bottle and shake well. Spray onto wood and wipe clean with a soft, dry cloth.

MOISTURE-RICH DUSTER

This recipe is nourishing for older, dry wood. But use it sparingly as too much oil left on the wood will attract more dust. Adjust the amount of linseed and essential oils needed based on how much surface area you are treating.

> scant ⅛ cup linseed oil
> 3 drops lemon or sweet orange essential oil

Combine ingredients in a small cup and stir to mix. Apply small amounts at a time to a dry cloth and rub well into wood. Wipe with a dry cloth to remove any oil residue.

WOOD POLISHES, WASHES, AND WAXES

You can make larger batches of any of these formulas and store in a recycled coffee can or glass jar with a screw-top lid. Just be sure to shake or stir before applying to the polishing cloth. Keeping an old toothbrush or small paintbrush in the can or jar is an easy and less messy way of getting the liquid polish onto the cloth.

HERBAL WOOD POLISH

This formula leaves a light herbal aroma.

> ¼ cup linseed oil
> 3 drops lavender or rosemary essential oil

Combine oils in a bowl. Apply a light layer of polish to wood with a brush or cloth. Rub into wood with a soft cloth, using circular motions. Wipe again with a dry cloth.

Lemon-Walnut Wood Polish

If making a larger quantity to store, use 15 drops lemon essential oil instead of the lemon juice.

> ⅛ cup walnut oil
> ⅛ cup linseed oil
> ¼ cup lemon juice

Combine all ingredients in a bowl (or clean coffee can with lid, if making in quantity). Apply a light layer of polish to wood with a brush or cloth. Rub into wood with a soft cloth, using circular motions. Wipe again with a dry cloth.

Carnauba and Lavender Wood Paste

Carnauba is the hardest wax available. Combined with oil, it is an excellent wood restorative.

> 2 tablespoons carnauba wax chips
> 1 cup linseed, almond, walnut, or olive oil
> 6 drops lavender essential oil

Combine carnauba and linseed oil in a double boiler. Heat slowly, stirring until completely melted. Remove from heat, add essential oil, and blend well. Pour into a glass or tin container and allow to cool completely before sealing. To use, spread the paste on wood with a soft, dry cloth using small, circular motions. Buff with a second dry cloth.

TRADITIONAL BEESWAX POLISH

This formula is used on quality wood pieces (especially antique furniture) that have been treated with a light penetrating finish; do not use on lacquered, painted, or unfinished surfaces. The formula calls for turpentine, but you can substitute a citrus peel–derived product called Plant Thinner, made by Auro Organics (available in some natural foods stores). If using turpentine, take extra care in handling and storing.

8	ounces unrefined beeswax, grated
2½	cups turpentine
2	cups water
½	cup lemon juice
2	ounces grated castile soap
15	drops essential oil of choice

1. Melt the beeswax slowly in a double boiler. When melted, remove from heat and carefully stir in the turpentine. Set aside.

2. In a medium saucepan, bring the water and lemon juice to a boil. Add the grated soap and stir until the soap melts. Allow this mixture to cool for 5 minutes.

3. Very slowly, pour the lemon juice mixture in a fine stream into the beeswax mixture, stirring constantly. Add the essential oil and blend well. Pour into a shallow glass jar or tin can and allow to cool completely before putting the lid on.

4. Dip a soft, dry cloth into the polish and spread a small amount on the wood surface; use small, circular motions. Wipe and buff with a second dry cloth.

Hardwood Floor Wash

Note: *If you have loose boards or wood tiles, hand wipe these areas with the wash. Excess liquid from the mop can get in the cracks and cause further buckling.*

> 1½ cups water
> 1½ cups vinegar
> 20 drops peppermint essential oil

Combine all ingredients in a spray bottle. Use sparingly, working on small sections of the floor. Dry mop the floor after washing.

Citrus-Scented Wood Floor Wax

In this formula, the lemon juice and essential oils clean while the beeswax and carnauba wax nourish.

> 1 cup linseed oil
> ¼ cup lemon juice
> 2 tablespoons grated beeswax
> 2 tablespoons carnauba wax
> 6 drops lemon essential oil
> 2 drops sweet orange essential oil
> lemon juice

Place linseed oil, ¼ cup lemon juice, and waxes in a double boiler over low heat. Stir constantly until completely melted and smooth. Add the essential oils. Remove from heat and pour the mixture into a clean coffee can and allow to harden. Once the wax has hardened, tap the sides of the can until the wax breaks free. Turn out the wax and gently rub it on the floor, like a crayon. Saturate a cloth with lemon juice, wring out, and rub the wax tracings well into the floor. Buff with a clean, dry cloth.

DOUBLE-NUT WOOD POLISH

This one smells almost good enough to eat! (But don't.)

> ¼ cup almond oil
> ⅛ cup walnut oil
> 4 drops pure vanilla extract

Combine all ingredients in a bowl. Apply a light layer of polish to wood with a brush or cloth. Rub into wood with a soft cloth, using circular motions. Wipe again with a dry cloth.

WOODSY WOOD FLOOR WAX

This formula leaves behind a nice shine and an earthy scent.

> 2 cups linseed oil
> ¼ cup carnauba wax
> 2 tablespoons beeswax
> ¼ cup lemon juice
> 8 drops patchouli essential oil
> 10 drops cedar essential oil
>   lemon juice

Combine linseed oil, waxes, and the ¼ cup lemon juice in a double boiler over low heat. Stir constantly until all the wax is melted. Add the essential oils and blend well. Remove from heat. Pour into a clean coffee can and allow to cool. Once the wax has hardened, tap the sides of the can until the wax breaks free. Turn out the wax and gently rub it on the floor, like a crayon. With a cloth that has been saturated with lemon juice and wrung out, rub the wax tracings well into the floor. Buff with a clean, dry cloth.

WAX REMOVER

This formula is for wood floors without a protective varnish finish.

> 2 cups warm vinegar
> ½ cup lemon juice
> ½ cup water
> 1 capful liquid castile soap
> 10 drops essential oil of choice

Combine all ingredients. Dampen a sponge mop or soft-bristled brush with the formula and apply to the floor in sections, using short strokes. Wipe each floor section dry with a towel or clean mop before moving on to the next.

SOLUTIONS FOR WOOD PROBLEMS

Black heel marks. These can be removed by rubbing 2 or 3 drops of cedar or eucalyptus essential oil over the mark with a soft cloth.

● ● ● ● ●

Burns. For burns that have not penetrated the wood surface but have just left a mark, rub with a thin paste of rottenstone (or cigarette ashes), linseed oil, and 2 or 3 drops of peppermint or tea tree essential oil. (*Note:* Tea tree oil is not recommended for dark wood.) If the burn has penetrated the wood surface, you may have to refinish the area.

Crayon. Wipe crayon marks with a few drops of cedar, peppermint, or tea tree essential oil mixed with a dab of toothpaste. (*Note:* Tea tree oil is not recommended for dark wood.) Wipe clean with a cloth moistened with vinegar.

* * * * *

Grease on floors. Immediately place ice cubes on top of the spill to harden and prevent the grease from seeping further into the wood. If a grease layer forms, it can be scraped off with a blunt object, such as a popsicle stick. If the wood is unfinished or has a penetrating finish, squirt some vegetable oil soap and a few drops of eucalyptus essential oil over the spill. Blot the stain repeatedly with clean paper towels or cotton cloths.

* * * * *

Grease on furniture. If grease is spilled or splattered on furniture, immediately cover the stain with salt to absorb as much grease as possible. Wait an hour and then vacuum or carefully brush away the salt with a dry cloth. If a grease stain remains, put a soft towel over the spot and press with a warm iron — but be careful not to scorch the wood! Keep shifting the towel around, or replace it with a fresh one to avoid redepositing grease on the wood.

* * * * *

Painted wood floors. Wood floors that have been painted can be cleaned with a solution of 2 teaspoons washing soda and 1 cup rosemary or sage tea (strained and cooled) mixed with a gallon of warm water.

Scratches. For light-colored woods, wet a soft cloth with equal parts of lemon juice and olive or vegetable oil and gently rub into the wood. Scratches on walnut can be treated with — what else? — a freshly shelled raw walnut. Darker woods, like mahogany, can be treated with a cloth dipped in equal amounts of warm water and vinegar. If the scratch remains, you can fill it in with a crayon or oil pastel pencil. Scratch marks on wood floors may be removed by gently rubbing in a circular motion with very fine steel wool moistened with a hard wax, such as Citrus-Scented Wood Floor Wax (page 97) or Woodsy Wood Floor Wax (page 98).

●　●　●　●　●

Water stains and rings. Leaking vases and flowerpots or condensation from cold drink glasses can leave bleached rings on wood surfaces. To treat these stains, first remove old polish by wiping with a soft cloth dipped in full-strength vinegar. Wipe thoroughly with a dry cloth. Then apply mayonnaise or linseed oil, working from the outside to the center of the spot. Leave the oil or mayonnaise for several hours and then buff with a cloth. You can also rub 2 to 4 drops of peppermint essential oil on the stain. Toothpaste is reputedly another cure for water rings on wood. Whatever method you use, remember to test on an inconspicuous spot first.

WALLS & CARPETING

IN THIS CHAPTER
Wall Cleaners & Disinfectants

Carpet Shampoos • Rug Deodorizers

Helpful Hints

There's no doubt about it: Dirt and germs are everywhere, under our feet and surrounding us on all sides. Hopefully, we don't think too much about this fact of life or we'd start to feel a bit antsy about sitting on the floor. It can even be said that we need a certain amount of germs in our life to remain healthy. But it's probably wise to draw the line at allowing an entire ecosystem from gaining a foothold in the carpeting. And who likes to look at dreary, stained walls?

Wallpaper and carpeting are really semipermanent fixtures. You can replace your living room drapes in a flash if you've grown tired of looking at the "same old thing." But can you say the same about your bathroom wallpaper or den carpeting? The cost of these accessories isn't a casual matter either; it can be quite an investment to carpet or wallpaper a large room. It makes good sense then to use safe, organic products to care for walls and carpeting. Not only are they better for you and the environment, but they will help to preserve the color and texture of wall coverings and carpet fibers.

KEEPING WALLS CLEAN

With three boys in our house, fingerprints on walls are just a part of life. The frequency of prints has lessened to a great extent in recent years, but when the boys were younger, the perpetual mural of hand- and fingerprints along the stairway could almost represent a daily growth chart. Of course, the kids loved earning a little money by taking on extra chores each Saturday, and cleaning off those fingerprints was one of the first tasks offered.

Walls painted with semigloss paint are the easiest to clean since they have a slick coating that doesn't absorb liquids. In fact, this is the preferred type of paint for kitchens, and especially for children's rooms, where a lot can happen to a wall. Latex can also be washed, but lightly. Scrubbing and repeated application of moisture may remove not only dirt and stains but the paint as well. The best way to clean painted walls is to use a solution of equal parts of vinegar and water. To a full spray bottle of solution add 6 to 10 drops of your favorite essential oil for grease-cutting power. Just make sure to use a clear or light essential oil on walls, such as eucalyptus, mint, or tea tree. (*Note:* Tea tree oil should be used on white walls only.)

Most wallpaper made today is washable, with some even being labeled as "scrubbable." Washable papers usually have a thin plastic film; scrubbable papers are either coated or impregnated with vinyl. In truth, you really can't "scrub" either one, nor should you use abrasive cleansers that could mar the paper's protective coating. The right way to clean wallpaper is to use small circular motions with a soapy cloth or sponge. The paper should then be wiped with a damp sponge and dried with a clean towel or cloth. If it becomes necessary to wash an area a second time, the paper must be allowed to dry thoroughly first. Overwetting wallpaper can cause the glue on the backing to dissolve, and soon your beautiful paper will be on the floor, not on your wall.

Wallpapered walls should be dusted frequently to reduce the risk of staining and streaking. This is especially true in the kitchen and bathroom, where hot water and steam can encourage a film to develop on dirty wallpaper. If you have a wall brush attachment with your vacuum cleaner, you can use it to dust your walls. If not, an old broom or mop handle with clean rags attached to one end will suffice.

Safe and Simple Wall Formulas

The following formulas will enable you to safely clean painted walls and wallpaper. If you have a stain removal issue and know that you have nonwashable wallpaper, consult the manufacturer or check with the store where it was purchased for cleaning recommendations. Regardless of what type of paper or paint covers your walls, always test a cleaning formula on a small area for a reaction before attempting to clean the entire surface.

ALL-PURPOSE CITRUS WALL CLEANER

This is a good general formula to safely clean wall surfaces.

    1 cup water
    ½ cup vinegar
    6 drops lemon, grapefruit, or orange
       essential oil

Combine all ingredients in a spray bottle. Shake vigorously before each use. Lightly spray the affected areas of your wall and wipe with a clean, damp sponge. If you're working on a stain and it's still visible after the area has completely air-dried, see the tips for cleaning walls on pages 107–108.

DISINFECTANT THYME FORMULA

This recipe is great for cleaning wall surfaces in a child's room, as well as light switches, the sides of the crib, or wherever little fingers tend to leave smudges and germs.

    1 cup water
    1 cup vinegar
    5 drops tea tree essential oil
    3 drops thyme essential oil

Combine all ingredients in a spray bottle. Lightly spray the affected areas of your wall and wipe with a clean, damp sponge. Give a final wipe to surfaces with a sponge or cloth moistened with plain water.

MINTY WALL CLEANSING PASTE ....

This cleanser is nonabrasive and will dissolve grease and fingerprints. It is recommended for use on washable papers or semigloss painted walls that are usually found in the kitchen, bathroom, and children's bedrooms. Note: The small amount of tea tree oil will not harm colored wallpaper.

> ¼ cup concentrated oil soap paste (available in natural food and hardware stores)
> 2 drops peppermint essential oil
> 2 drops spearmint essential oil
> 2 drops tea tree essential oil

Put the soap paste in a short, widemouthed glass jar, such as a clean baby food jar. Add the essential oils and blend well. It will have the consistency of jelly. Dip a damp cloth into the soap paste and squish the cloth between your fingers to make suds. Apply to wallpaper; rinse with another clean, damp cloth or sponge. Follow up with a dry cloth or towel.

HELPFUL HINTS
FOR CLEANING WALLS

Always clean walls by working from the bottom up to the ceiling. This advice may seem odd to you, but there is good reason for it. If you've ever tried the reverse — cleaning from top to bottom — then you've probably experienced those drip lines that travel down the wall and stay there. Those streaks of cleaning product have been working ahead of you and are very difficult to get rid of. This problem is eliminated if you take the floor-to-ceiling approach.

Stains and spots on nonwashable papers may be dealt with by rubbing a pencil eraser or art gum over them. The same applies to pencil marks. Or rub a freshly cut rhubarb stalk over the stain and wipe with a damp cloth. Test both methods on a small area out of view first.

* * * * *

Got a grease stain? Tear or cut a paper towel into four squares. To one square apply 1 or 2 drops of eucalyptus essential oil and allow it to dry. Using an iron on a low setting, press the oil-treated paper towel square against the grease stain for a few seconds. Then immediately press a clean paper towel square against the stain. Repeat this procedure with the remaining paper towel squares. If the grease stain remains, wait a few hours and apply a thick paste of cream of tartar, baking soda, and enough water to hold everything together. Brush the paste away when it has dried to a powder. If both of these methods fail, consider repainting or start shopping for new wallpaper.

* * * * *

Crayon scribbling on painted walls or wallpaper can be tough to tackle. Fortunately, most crayons are washable today, but the nonwashable type are still around. Try the methods described above for removing grease spots. If the crayon mark endures, and if it's on a painted surface, scrub (yes, scrub) the area with liquid castile soap and 1 or 2 drops of orange essential oil. I wouldn't try this on wallpaper (unless you think yours might hold up), but you should be able to remove it from a painted wall without causing too much damage. A "weathered" look on the wall is better than waxy lines of color.

* * * * *

Food stains, especially spaghetti sauce, always seem to make impossible leaps from the simmering pot on the stove to the kitchen wall several feet away (and onto everything in between). If wiped right away there's usually no problem. But we never seem to notice these stains until we go looking for them, usually before a party or important entertaining event. If the wall is covered with washable paint or wallpaper, your task is less daunting; just wipe it with the All-Purpose Citrus Wall Cleaner (see page 105). If the wall is covered with latex paint or nonwashable wallpaper you may have more trouble. Carefully scrape off as much as you can with a blunt object or dull knife. If a noticeable stain remains, place 3 drops of eucalyptus essential oil on a cotton ball and then dip it in baking soda. Dab the stain with cotton ball a few times and then rub until the stain disappears.

DEEP CLEANING THE CARPETS?

To a lot of people, the term "deep cleaning" seems to conjure up a vision of a sea of foaming suds and water whisking away dirt from "way under." All that soapy sloshing must really get a carpet clean, right? Wrong. Too much soap and water will leave a residue in the carpet that acts like a magnet for dirt. And getting the backing of the carpet wet only creates a pool for the dirt (and stains) to collect in, not to mention promoting the potential for mildew and shrinkage of the carpet. So the first rule of carpet cleaning in terms of cleaning products is "less is more."

If you've ever steamed or shampooed your carpet by machine and have had to empty the collection tank, then you're already aware of how much gunk lives in the carpet fibers. In addition to minute pieces of sand and dead skin, there's a host of nasty critters such as mites and, if you have pets, fleas. All of these will ruin carpet fibers if given free reign. Frequent vacuuming (at least once each week) will displace these critters and their food source at the same time. Heavy traffic areas, such as hallways, stairs, and foyers, can be swept with a broom or a carpet sweeper before vacuuming. This helps to lift the nap of the carpet and bring soil to the surface for easier removal.

Do-It-Yourself Carpet Remedies

Just like the little fingerprints on our walls, footprints and spills of uncertain origin are not strangers to our wall-to-wall carpeting. Exercise the familiar "please, wipe your feet" as often as you will, but energy-driven kids in muddy sneakers often forget to pause at the doormat. This section offers some safe herbal and alternative solutions for cleaning carpets, as well as tips for treating some pretty sticky messes.

ROSEMARY–LAVENDER CARPET SHAMPOO

This recipe makes enough for a 10' x 13' room. If you can't find soap flakes, you may use ¼ cup of borax instead, but test the outcome of this substitution on a small area first.

- 2 cups baking soda
- ½ cup soap flakes
- 20 drops lavender essential oil
- 8 drops rosemary essential oil
- ½ cup vinegar
- 2 cups warm water

1. Sweep the carpet to be cleaned with a broom or carpet sweeper to loosen dirt, then vacuum the entire area.

2. Combine the baking soda and soap flakes in a plastic bowl. Add the essential oils and mix well, breaking up any clumps with a fork. Sprinkle the mixture on the carpet.

3. Add the vinegar to the warm water in a bucket or pail. Dip a clean sponge mop into the bucket and squeeze out as much excess liquid as you can. Gently go over the carpet with the sponge mop, working in sections. Wait at least an hour and then vacuum again.

PEPPERMINT FOAM CARPET SHAMPOO

This formula is great for cleaning heavy traffic areas.

- 3 cups water
- ¾ cup vegetable-based liquid soap
- 10 drops peppermint essential oil

Mix all ingredients in a blender. Rub the foam into soiled areas with a damp sponge. Let dry thoroughly and then vacuum.

SIMPLE RUG & CARPET DEODORIZER

Pets and bare feet can cause a rather "funky" smell. This formula leaves your carpets looking and smelling fresh again.

- 1 cup borax
- 1 cup baking soda
- ½ cup cornmeal
- 10 drops juniper essential oil
- 5 drops cypress essential oil

Combine the dry ingredients in a plastic bowl. Add essential oils and mix well, breaking up clumps. Sprinkle the mixture over carpet and wait several hours, overnight if possible, before vacuuming.

HERBAL RUG RESTORER

Alum and vinegar combine to clean and lift carpet fibers. The essential oils leave a fresh herbal scent. Note: For spot treatment, rub a little baking soda into soiled areas. Let dry and brush clean with a soft-bristled brush; follow with Rug Restorer. Use gloves if your hands will be coming in contact with the cleaner.

- ½ gallon hot water
- ½ cup alum
- ¼ cup vinegar
- 8 drops rosemary essential oil
- 3 drops lemon essential oil

Combine all ingredients in a pail or bucket. Fill a second bucket with hot water for rinsing. Dip a clean sponge mop into the vinegar solution, squeeze out excess liquid, and wipe over carpet in sections. Rinse the mop in the second bucket between cleaning sections and squeeze out excess water. Repeat until all of the carpet has been cleaned.

Try this excellent formula to rid yourself of those pesky little critters. It may seem wasteful, but it's best to get rid of the vacuum cleaner bag after this treatment to prevent reinfestation of fleas.

2½ cups baking soda
10 drops sweet orange essential oil
10 drops citronella essential oil
8 drops peppermint or spearmint essential oil
6 drops lemon or lemon balm essential oil

Vacuum carpet well. Combine all ingredients in a plastic container and sprinkle on carpet. Wait at least one hour before vacuuming again.

HELPFUL HINTS FOR CLEANING CARPETING

Spills should be cleaned up as soon as possible. Always blot a stain with towels or cloths to absorb excess liquid. Rubbing the stain vigorously can cause further penetration of the spill into the carpet fibers and backing.

· · · · ·

Be careful not to saturate a carpet when using liquid cleaners, or even water. If the backing gets wet, the invading stain will have a safe place to hide and it will be much more difficult to remove.

· · · · ·

Most food stains can be safely removed with a solution of vinegar and a bit of dishwashing soap.

You can add a few drops of essential oil to the vinegar first if you like.

* * * * *

Blood stains and spots should be blotted with cold water or club soda. If the stain doesn't come out completely, use a cloth moistened with cold water and 2 drops eucalyptus essential oil.

* * * * *

Sprinkle mud stains with salt or baking soda. Wait 30 minutes, then vacuum.

* * * * *

For ink stains, first cover with cream of tartar. Then take a fresh lemon wedge and squeeze a few drops of juice over the cream of tartar. Using the flesh of the lemon, gently go over the spot a few times. Brush away the powder and blot with a damp sponge.

* * * * *

Urine stains should first be blotted with paper towels to absorb as much of the liquid as possible. With a sponge, apply a solution of ¼ cup vinegar, 1 teaspoon dishwashing soap, and 8 to 10 drops of peppermint or eucalyptus essential oil; wait 20 minutes. (The vinegar and essential oils will help to sanitize the soiled area and remove any odor.) Blot the stained area again using a clean, damp towel. *Note:* Vinegar can sometimes slightly bleach dark-colored carpets. Test this formula on an inconspicuous area first.

CLEANING
METALS

IN THIS CHAPTER

Stain & Buildup Removers • Specialty Formulas

Tarnish Removers

Metal polishes may contain one or more strong acids that quickly dissolve tarnish. These acids can also burn human skin. Hydrofluoric acid, used in some rust removers and aluminum polishes, is probably the most hazardous. If it gets on your skin it continues to penetrate until it permeates the bone. Of course, protective gloves should be worn when handling such chemicals but, in spite of any precautions taken, does this sound like something you want to put your hands in? Worse yet, do you want to use it on utensils and vessels that are used to serve food?

REMOVING METAL STAINS AND BUILDUP

Many people are convinced that a caustic commercial polish is necessary to adequately perform the task of removing rust and tarnish from metals. But you probably already have the ingredients readily available in your kitchen or garden to do the job safely and to do it well. You may not have the instant results that might be achieved with a commercial polish, but you will get good results if you allow some time for the formulas suggested here to work. Besides, rust and tarnish do not develop overnight, why expect them to disappear in a moment?

Aluminum

Aluminum is the most abundant metal found in the earth's crust, but does not occur as a free metal; it is usually found as aluminum silicate or mixed with other minerals such as iron, calcium, and magnesium. Since the expense of extracting the aluminum from these silicate mixtures is too great, bauxite, an impure hydrated oxide, is the common source of commercial aluminum.

When in contact with air, new aluminum quickly forms a durable oxide layer that protects it from corrosion. This is why aluminum products never rust or tarnish. Aluminum is, however, highly reactive, and two commonly used ingredients in homemade metal cleaners should never be used on it: baking soda and washing soda.

Since aluminum resists corrosion and tarnish, superficial stains are the only problems to contend with. Spruce up your aluminum by cleaning with one of these methods:

- In a sink or a plastic tub, mix 2 cups of boiled water, 1 cup of vinegar, and 1 teaspoon of any citrus essential oil. Place aluminum items in the solution and let soak for an hour or more. Rinse and dry well before storing.
- Combine 2 tablespoons cornstarch, 2 tablespoons alum, 5 drops of lemon or orange essential oil, and enough water to make a thick paste. While wearing gloves, rub onto metal until clean. Rinse and dry well.
- Make a paste of ¼ cup vinegar and 2 tablespoons cream of tartar; add 2 to 4 drops of a citrus essential oil, if desired. Spread the paste on the metal and rub with your glove-protected fingers until it is clean. Rinse and dry well.
- For utensils, place 1 cup of sliced rhubarb in 2 cups of water (or enough water to submerge the items) in a pot. Simmer for 30 minutes. Rinse utensils in cool water and dry. *Note:* Fresh or canned tomato slices can be used in place of the rhubarb.

Brass

Brass is an alloy of copper and zinc. Most brass items acquired in recent years will have a lacquer finish to retard tarnish. You can maintain the shine of these items with a weekly dusting and an occasional bath in warm, sudsy water. Never use hot water to clean brass items or the lacquer finish

You need to be careful when cleaning antique brass items so that you don't disturb the aged coloring of the piece, or what is referred to as it's patina. The best way to clean these pieces is first with a bath in warm, soapy water to remove filmy dirt and grease. Then polish with a soft cloth moistened with linseed oil. If you have a very old or delicate piece and are not sure how to approach cleaning it, you may want to consult with an expert, such as an antiques dealer, refinisher, or museum curator. Brass andirons should be cleaned with extra-fine steel wool or emery cloth, rubbing the metal in one direction only.

may begin to peel away from the metal. After cleaning, you can polish the brass to a shine with a bit of olive oil, which will help to resist tarnish.

Older pieces of brass will oxidize over time and become tarnished, developing a greenish tinge. Here are a few ways to restore brass to its original beauty:

- Dissolve 4 drops of any citrus essential oil and 2 teaspoons of salt in 1 cup of vinegar. Add just enough all-purpose flour to make a thick paste. Smear the paste onto the brass and rub with a dry sponge. Let the paste completely dry, then rinse in warm water. Dry and polish to a shine.

- Combine ¼ cup vinegar, ¼ cup Worcestershire sauce, 3 drops lemon essential oil, and 3 drops grapefruit seed extract. Using a soft sponge, apply this solution to the metal and rub well. If the item is very tarnished, let it soak for 30 minutes or more in this solution. Then rinse and dry thoroughly.

- Soak your brass pieces in 1 cup of warm water and 1 cup of milk (or more for larger pieces — just use equal parts of milk and water). Milk contains lactic acid, a natural solvent.
- Make a paste of ¼ cup lemon juice, 4 to 6 drops of orange or lemon essential oil, and 2 to 3 tablespoons cream of tartar. Rub the paste on with your fingers (wear protective gloves) using small circular motions. Let the paste dry. Then rinse and dry with a cloth.

Bronze

Bronze is also an alloy of copper, but unlike brass, it is combined with almost any other metal but zinc. Like brass, however, solid bronze pieces are often lacquered to prevent tarnishing. Good quality bronze pieces, especially those displayed outdoors, develop a lovely patina as they age. This look is often duplicated in art and reproduction pieces. Since this "weathered" effect is highly desirable in bronze, regular dusting and light polishing with a soft cloth are generally all you need to do. A soft brush can be used on items that have been neglected for a time. If you want a high polish on a bronze item, you can wipe it clean and then shine it with a cloth dipped in a liquid wax.

Bronze is also susceptible to "bronze disease," characterized by isolated spots of corrosion and light green patches. This is caused by exposure to chlorides, sulfides, or excessive moisture. Usually, this "disease" can be remedied by bathing the piece in boiled distilled water, changing the water several times during the process. It may be necessary to soak the item for several days. You can also use hot vinegar and salt, or even hot buttermilk. If these treatments don't cure the problem, you'll need to call an expert.

To clean dirt and grease from bronze, pull on protective gloves and rub the item vigorously with a cloth moistened with a solution of 1 cup vinegar, ⅛ cup grapefruit juice, and 6 drops pine or cedar essential oil. Rinse in warm water and dry completely with a soft, clean towel.

Cast Iron

My father is a native of Alabama, where cornbread is a staple and often made in a cast iron skillet. When I was growing up, I recall such a skillet in our kitchen and when it wasn't being used it was stored in the oven. One day, I decided to give the pan a good scrubbing with soap and water and left it to air-dry in the dish rack. When I returned to put the pan away I puzzled over how it became dirty looking again. In fact, it looked worse than before! My mistake, of course, was in letting the pan air-dry and form rust.

Cast iron will oxidize and rust if not kept completely dry at all times. It must also be "seasoned" with oil to form a protective barrier and prevent oxidation. When you acquire a new piece of cast iron, you need to clean it with a mild soap and fine steel wool and dry it by hand immediately. Then the interior should be wiped with a bit of vegetable oil and the pan set in a low oven (250°F) for two hours. After the pan has cooled, wipe it out and wash once more, taking care to dry it thoroughly. Now the pan is properly seasoned and ready to use.

After each use, cast iron should be wiped and quickly washed and dried. Another application of oil is needed before storing the pan. Cast iron pans should not be stored with the lids in place, as this can trap moisture. It's also a good idea to place a paper towel inside the pan when storing to absorb excess moisture. If it becomes necessary to scour cast iron to remove cooked-on foods, it will be necessary to reseason the pan.

Chrome

Chrome is a hard metal with a whitish-blue appearance. Its durability and shine make it suitable for plating other metals to extend the life of the object. Chrome, or chromium, is frequently found on appliances such as toasters, ovens, refrigerators, faucets, vehicles — even golf clubs. If kept free of grease and sticky grime, chrome can last a very long time. Here are some tips for keeping chrome in tip-top shape:

- Never use an abrasive cleaner on chrome that may scratch or pit the surface.
- To safely clean chrome, apply club soda or vinegar with a soft cloth. Dry to a shine with a dry cloth.
- To remove burned-on grease from chrome, clean with 3 to 6 drops of undiluted eucalyptus or peppermint essential oil (wear protective gloves). Wipe dry with a clean cloth.

■ For rust stains, first clean with a rag and a few drops of eucalyptus or peppermint essential oil. Then rub the stains with a small piece of crumpled aluminum foil, shiny side out. Wipe well with a soft cloth moistened with 3 to 6 drops of essential oil and 1 tablespoon of jojoba or almond oil (mix the essential oils into the jojoba or almond oil first).

Copper

Decorative copper items are usually coated with lacquer to preserve the finish; they should never be polished. Only regular dusting and periodic washing are necessary. Copper cookware and utensils, on the other hand, may need special handling to remove any factory-applied lacquer. Follow the manufacturer's directions; if there aren't any instructions included, the copper pieces should be placed in 2 gallons of boiling water and 1½ cups washing soda. Let them soak until you are able to peel away the lacquer.

Stainless steel pots and pans often have copper bottoms for better distribution of heat, but high temperatures can damage them. Never scour copper bottoms with steel wool or an abrasive cleanser. If tarnishing occurs, use equal amounts of salt, flour, and vinegar to make a polishing paste.

To clean and remove tarnish from copper pots and utensils, try one of these tricks:

■ Cut a lime or lemon in half, sprinkle with salt, and rub over the copper. If you don't have any fresh lemons or limes on hand, you can use lemon juice or 1 teaspoon of any citrus essential oil mixed with 2 tablespoons water instead. Apply this solution to a damp sponge that has been sprinkled with salt. Nothing can be easier than this!

■ Make a paste of 1 cup vinegar, 5 drops citrus essential oil, 1¼ cups all-purpose flour, and ½ cup salt. Spread the paste on your copper pieces and let stand for a few hours or overnight. Then rinse, dry, and polish with a bit of oil to prevent further tarnishing.

■ Mix ½ cup ketchup with 2 tablespoons cream of tartar. Spread on the copper and let stand for an hour. Rinse in soapy water and then in clean water. Dry thoroughly.

COPPER CAUTIONS

Copper can also be vulnerable to "bronze disease." Follow the suggestions given on page 118–119 for cleaning bronze to tackle this problem.

Pots or bowls with copper interiors cannot be used for preparing or storing acidic foods such as fruits, tomatoes, or anything containing vinegar. These foods can react with copper to form toxic compounds.

Pewter

Antique pewter is an alloy of lead and tin. Old pewter develops a dark patina over time that looks beautiful, but due to the lead content, such pieces cannot be used to prepare or serve foods. Most pewter pieces made today are tarnish resistant, being composed of roughly 90 percent tin and 10 percent copper or antimony. This combination of metals retains its original color and is lead-free, but is not as durable and is vulnerable to dents and scratches. Some imitation pewter pieces are made from aluminum. To be safe, check the manufacturer's instructions for the appropriate care and cleaning of individual items. Try these quick fixes for your pewter pieces:

- Pewter can be cleaned by rubbing with wet cabbage leaves or freshly cut leaf wedges.
- Revive dull pewter with a paste made from ¼ cup fine rottenstone, 2 teaspoons linseed oil, and 4 drops peppermint or wintergreen essential oil. (*Note:* Be careful not to overdo it when cleaning antique pewter — it's supposed to have a dark color due to its lead content.)
- You can also clean pewter pieces with a solution of 1 teaspoon salt dissolved in 1 cup vinegar. Add 4 drops essential oil of choice and enough all-purpose flour to make a paste. Rub onto the metal with glove-protected fingertips. Rinse well and dry thoroughly.

Silver

Silver has many seemingly innocent enemies. Rubber, for instance, not only promotes tarnishing when in contact with silver, it can actually corrode the finish. Using rubber gloves while cleaning silver is definitely not a good idea. Likewise, avoid storing silver in rubber-lined cabinets or storage boxes. Even binding silver pieces together with rubber bands can prove detrimental.

Other substances that have a negative impact on silver include olives, eggs, salad dressing, fruit juices, vinegar, and salt. And, believe it or not, flowers should never be placed in a silver vase unless it is lined with a glass or plastic container first. As cut flowers decompose they release an acid that can permanently etch silver finishes.

Sterling silver is actually an alloy of approximately 92.5 percent silver and 7.5 percent copper; plated silver has a layer of silver electroplated over another metal. All silver readily oxidizes and responds to hand polishing for the best sheen and patina. The best course of action to deter tarnishing of silver flatware is to use it often, but never allow food to stand. If you can't wash it right away, rinse off any food residue until you can give your flatware a proper cleaning. (*Note:* Some decorative pieces may be lacquered; care should be taken to avoid contact with hot water.) When silver is not in use, it should be stored rolled up in a flannel cloth.

If you put your silver flatware in the dishwasher, it's best to hand-dry the items instead of letting them go through the heated drying cycle. Also, it's important to separate silver flatware from other pieces, such as stainless steel, in the silverware basket of your dishwasher to avoid scratching or possible chemical reactions with other materials.

If you have a problem with tarnish, here are a couple of formulas to try:

■ **Easy Tarnish Remover.** Place silver pieces in a sink or pan filled with water. Add 2 tablespoons cream of tartar and a few strips of aluminum foil. Let the silver soak for an hour or until tarnish free. (If the silver is badly tarnished, you may notice an odor like rotten eggs. This is due to a chemical reaction causing the release of hydrogen sulfide gas. This gas isn't concentrated enough to be harmful, but it might be a good idea to open a window if it occurs.) Rinse silver and hand-dry all pieces with a soft cloth.

■ **Instant Tarnish Remover.** Squeeze some ordinary toothpaste into a small bowl and add 3 to 5 drops of peppermint or spearmint essential oil. Rub this mixture with your fingertips onto the silver. As the tarnish is removed, the toothpaste mixture will turn grayish. Rinse the silver well and hand-dry thoroughly before storing. Since gloves shouldn't be worn while cleaning silver, wash hands well when finished. If your skin begins to itch while using the cleaner, rinse well.

WHAT ABOUT GOLD?

Gold is a soft metal and can easily be scratched by abrasives. The safest way to clean gold is with a paste of 1 teaspoon liquid castile soap and 1 tablespoon baking soda. Using your fingertips, gently rub the paste onto the item. Rinse in warm water and dry thoroughly with a soft cloth or towel.

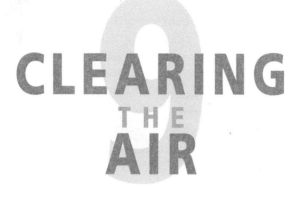

CLEARING THE AIR

In medieval Europe, herbs and spices played an important role in the maintenance of the household, not only for their culinary qualities, but also for their ability to mask unpleasant odors caused by poor hygiene and unsanitary conditions.

Today, although we may no longer be plagued by insufficient sanitation, we have a new challenge to face from modern household materials: Ordinary carpeting, furniture, and painted surfaces all produce toxic vapors such as VOCs (volatile organic compounds), trichlorethylene, and formaldehyde. Obviously, unless we choose to live in a tent, we cannot escape or avoid every contaminant found in building materials. But we can greatly reduce their impact on our health by purifying the air to minimize their presence in the home. How? By developing a green thumb.

CLEAN AND GREEN

You may recall from high school biology that plants are involved in a process called photosynthesis. During this process, plants continuously take in carbon dioxide and other airborne toxins to produce oxygen. Bingo! You've got instant air filtration. In fact, it has been estimated that 15 to 20 spider plants will effectively detoxify a home of less than 2,000 square feet. Of course, almost any type of plant will help to do the same.

If you're wondering where you are going to put all these plants, consider hanging baskets, plant stands that can hold several plants at a time, or even mini gardens on windowsills. If natural lighting is a problem, artificial lighting, such as grow lights, will keep your living air purifiers healthy. If you have "little ones" or pets, be sure to keep plants — especially poisonous ones — out of their reach.

Some common plants that purify air are:

- Spider plant, also known as airplane plant (*Chlorophytum comosum* 'vittatum')
- Golden pothos *(Epipremnum aureum)*
- Peace lily (*Spathiphyllum* species)
- Fern (*Pteris* species and *Nephrolepis* species)
- Chinese evergreen (*Aglaonema modestum* 'Silver Queen')
- Weeping fig *(Ficus benjamina)*

Herbs also filter the air, and many can easily be grown indoors year-round. Basil, thyme, oregano, sage, rosemary, mints, and geraniums are just some herbs that not only help to clean the air but offer aromatic properties of their own, not to mention adding flavor to your favorite dishes.

POTPOURRI

Potpourri gets its name from a marriage of the French words *pot* and *pourri* (to rot) — collectively, "rotting pot." One modern definition of potpourri is a literary or musical medley; for our purposes, it's a harmonic composition of botanical fragrances.

There is essentially no end to the different types of potpourri that you can create. All successful dried formulas require a "fixative," which captures the aromatic oils from flowers, spices, and herbs when blended together. Common fixatives include orrisroot (the dried, ground rhizome of the iris plant), oakmoss, calamus root (sweet flag), gum benzoin, frankincense, cinnamon sticks, and patchouli. Fixatives can also take the form of "woody" material, such as pinecones, milkweed pods, and cedar shavings or chips. Some craft stores carry a fixative made from dried corncobs.

The base of a potpourri is made of dried aromatic herbs and plants, and may include flowers, stems, and leaves. Spices such as cloves, ginger, and nutmeg are also used in making potpourri blends. Fragrant herbal essential oils add concentrated aroma to potpourri and are easily obtainable. Pieces of dried bark, berries, fruit peels, and unusual seedpods are not only attractive, but also act as fixatives and help to preserve the scent. Bear in mind, however, that trial and error is often necessary to achieve the right balance in a potpourri, especially in its application. For instance, some potpourri ingredients may smell strong in the dry form, but are lost to other ingredients that prevail when simmered in water.

It isn't necessary to add a fixative to a potpourri intended to be simmered unless you desire additional fragrance. Do not add benzoin to a simmering potpourri; although it has a nice fragrance in dried form, it is rather unpleasant when simmered. The key to making interesting potpourri blends lies in your desire to experiment, but many variations are offered here to spark your imagination.

A MIDSUMMER'S EVE

This outdoorsy potpourri may be added to pillows and sachets or set out in a dish or bowl.

½ cup purple basil
½ cup chamomile
½ cup marjoram
¼ cup yarrow (white or yellow)
¼ cup juniper berries
¼ cup oakmoss
2 tablespoons gum benzoin
2 tablespoons mace
1 teaspoon grated orange peel
15 drops cedar essential oil

Combine all ingredients in a glass jar and stir with a spoon until well blended. Cap the jar and leave it in a place free of drafts, direct sunlight, and extreme temperatures. Gently shake the jar once a day for 4 to 6 weeks, or until you feel that the fragrance has fully developed.

Elegant Romance

A lovely potpourri, Elegant Romance may be simmered in a pan of hot water on the stove, added to pillows and sachets, or set out in a dish or bowl. Note: Sandalwood is highly valued in the perfume industry for its rich scent. Because it is extracted from the roots of a tree that can take up to 75 years to reach maturity, it is not readily renewable and is a bit expensive. Please use it sparingly.

> 1 cup rose petals
> 1 cup lavender buds
> 1 cup rose geranium leaves
> ½ cup lemon verbena leaves
> ½ cup powdered orrisroot
> 10 drops vanilla fragrance oil
> 8 drops sandalwood essential oil

Combine all ingredients in a glass jar and stir with a spoon until well blended. Cap the jar and leave it in a place free of drafts, direct sunlight, and extreme temperatures. Gently shake the jar once a day for 4 to 6 weeks, or until you feel that the fragrance has fully developed.

Spring Fresh

This strongly fragrant potpourri may be simmered in a pan of hot water on the stove, added to pillows and sachets, or set out in a dish or bowl.

> ½ cup rosemary leaves
> ½ cup peppermint or spearmint leaves
> ½ cup eucalyptus leaves, torn
> ¼ cup thyme leaves
> ¼ cup whole cloves
> 2 teaspoons grated lemon peel
> 1 teaspoon grated orange peel

Combine all ingredients in a glass jar and stir with a spoon until well blended. Cap the jar and leave it in a place free of drafts, direct sunlight, and extreme temperatures. Gently shake the jar once a day for 4 to 6 weeks, or until you feel that the fragrance has fully developed.

GARDEN MEMORIES

This colorful blend may be added to pillows and sachets or set out in a dish or bowl.

1 cup calendula flowers
1 cup statice
1 cup cornflowers
1 cup snapdragons
½ cup rose petals
½ cup sunflower petals
½ cup marigolds
½ cup rose hips
½ cup juniper berries
¼ cup cedar chips
¼ cup anise, ground
2 cinnamon sticks, crushed

Combine all ingredients in a glass jar and stir with a spoon until well blended. Cap the jar and leave it in a place free of drafts, direct sunlight, and extreme temperatures. Gently shake the jar once a day for 4 to 6 weeks, or until you feel that the fragrance has fully developed.

COUNTRY ROADS

Simmer this potpourri in a pan of hot water on the stove, or add it to pillows and sachets. You can also set it out in a pretty dish or bowl.

> 2 cups dried apple slices
> 1 cup bay leaves
> 1 cup sage
> ½ cup gingerroot, chopped but not peeled
> ½ cup whole cloves
> 8 1-inch cinnamon sticks

Combine all ingredients in a glass jar and stir with a spoon until well blended. Cap the jar and leave it in a place free of drafts, direct sunlight, and extreme temperatures. Gently shake the jar once a day for 4 to 6 weeks, or until you feel that the fragrance has fully developed.

EXOTIC BLEND

Don't simmer this blend; instead, add it to pillows and sachets or set out in an unusual dish or bowl.

> ½ cup jasmine flowers
> ¼ cup lemon verbena
> ¼ cup lavender
> ¼ cup sweet woodruff
> ¼ cup fennel leaves
> 2 teaspoons coriander peel
> 2 teaspoons gingerroot

Combine all ingredients in a glass jar and stir with a spoon until well blended. Cap the jar and leave it in a place free of drafts, direct sunlight, and extreme temperatures. Gently shake the jar once a day for 4 to 6 weeks.

Parlor Potpourri

When it's ready, transfer the potpourri into small decorative containers and place on tables, shelves, or any other place it will be visually appreciated.

¼ cup whole cloves
¼ cup allspice berries
¼ cup brown sugar
¼ cup bay leaves, crushed
¾ cup noniodized salt
1 cup rose petals
1 cup hydrangea petals
½ cup rose geranium leaves, dried
½ cup lavender flowers
½ cup rosemary sprigs, dried and crumbled
¼ cup bay leaves, crushed
¼ cup orrisroot
2 tablespoons cognac

1. Combine the cloves, allspice, brown sugar, bay leaves, and salt in a bowl.

2. In a separate bowl, mix the remaining ingredients except the cognac. Place some of this mixture in a widemouthed jar or crock and sprinkle with some of the salt mixture. Continue alternating layers in this manner, ending with a layer of the salt mixture.

3. Sprinkle the cognac over all and place a heavy rock on top to weigh the mixture down. Tightly seal the jar or crock.

4. Stir this mixture once a day for 4 to 6 weeks, replacing the weight each time. If the mixture dries out, add a bit more cognac.

ORANGE DELIGHT

This spicy potpourri may be simmered in a pan of hot water on the stove, added to pillows and sachets, or set out in a dish or bowl.

> 2 cups orange peel, cut into small strips
> 1 cup marigold flower heads
> 1 cup dried apple, cubed
> ½ cup whole cloves
> ½ cup cinnamon chips
> ½ cup calamus root
> 10 drops sweet orange essential oil

Combine all ingredients in a glass jar and stir with a spoon until well blended. Cap the jar and leave it in a place free of drafts, direct sunlight, and extreme temperatures. Gently shake the jar once a day for 4 to 6 weeks, or until you feel that the fragrance has fully developed.

SINFUL SEDUCTION

Add this potpourri to pillows and sachets or set out in a dish or bowl. Note: Tonka beans, members of the pea family, are flavorless yet contain a strong vanilla-like scent. You can find them in health food stores.

> 1 cup jasmine flowers
> 1 cup lemon verbena leaves
> ½ cup chopped gingerroot
> ½ cup clary sage leaves, crushed
> 2 tonka beans
> 1 vanilla bean, chopped into small pieces
> 1 tablespoon sandalwood chips
> 1 teaspoon cumin seed
> 20 drops patchouli essential oil

Combine all ingredients in a glass jar and stir with a spoon until well blended. Cap the jar and leave it in a place free of drafts, direct sunlight, and extreme temperatures. Gently shake the jar once a day for 4 to 6 weeks, or until you feel that the fragrance has fully developed.

ENCHANTED HUMMINGBIRD

This potpourri contains some noted "hummingbird flowers." It may be added to pillows and sachets or set out in a dish or bowl.

> 1 cup magnolia flowers
> 1 cup rose hips
> 1 cup bee balm blossoms
> 1 cup lemon verbena
> ½ cup calendula flowers
> ¼ cup grated orange peel
> ¼ cup grated tangerine peel
> 2 tablespoons orrisroot
> 10 drops rose geranium essential oil
> 10 drops bergamot essential oil

Combine all ingredients in a glass jar and stir with a spoon until well blended. Cap the jar and leave it in a place free of drafts, direct sunlight, and extreme temperatures. Gently shake the jar once a day for 4 to 6 weeks, or until you feel that the fragrance has fully developed.

WOODLAND BREEZES

You can use this potpourri to stuff pillows and sachets, or display it in an attractive dish or bowl.

>   1 cup whole sage leaves
>   1 cup red nasturtium blossoms
>   1 cup evening primrose flowers
>   1 cup cedar chips
>   ½ cup clary sage leaves
>   ½ cup oakmoss
>   ¼ cup angelica root, chopped
>   25 drops patchouli essential oil

Combine all ingredients in a glass jar and stir with a spoon until well blended. Cap the jar and leave it in a place free of drafts, direct sunlight, and extreme temperatures. Gently shake the jar once a day for 4 to 6 weeks, or until you feel that the fragrance has fully developed.

MORNING DEW

A light, fresh blend, this potpourri may be added to pillows and sachets or set out in a dish or bowl.

>   1 cup lemon balm leaves and flowers
>   1 cup marigold blossoms
>   1 cup peppermint leaves
>   ½ cup chamomile flowers
>   ½ cup lemon thyme leaves
>   ¼ cup grated grapefruit peel
>   ¼ cup grated lemon peel
>   2 tablespoons coriander
>   1 tablespoon orrisroot
>   15 drops bergamot essential oil

Combine all ingredients in a glass jar and stir with a spoon until well blended. Cap the jar and leave it in a place free of drafts, direct sunlight, and extreme temperatures. Gently shake the jar once a day for 4 to 6 weeks, or until you feel that the fragrance has fully developed.

MULBERRY MADNESS

Displaying this potpourri in a bowl or dish will catch the attention of guests. You can also add the blend to pillows or sachets.

> 3 cups rose petals and leaves
> 1 cup juniper berries
> 1 cup hibiscus flowers
> ½ cup bay leaves, crushed
> ¼ cup star anise
> 2 tablespoons orrisroot
> 15 drops mulberry fragrance (liquid; available in craft stores)

Combine all ingredients in a glass jar and stir with a spoon until well blended. Cap the jar and leave it in a place free of drafts, direct sunlight, and extreme temperatures. Gently shake the jar once a day for 4 to 6 weeks, or until you feel that the fragrance has fully developed.

NICE 'N' SPICY

Nice 'n' Spicy is a great simmering blend, but it also can be added to pillows and sachets or displayed in a dish or bowl. Always use sandalwood oil sparingly, as the tree it is extracted from is endangered.

> 1 cup anise hyssop
> 1 cup fennel leaves
> ½ cup pineapple-scented sage
> ¼ cup grated orange peel
> 2 tablespoons aniseed, ground
> 1 tablespoon coriander
> 1 teaspoon caraway seeds
> 10 drops sandalwood essential oil
> 5 drops vanilla essential oil

Combine all ingredients in a glass jar and stir with a spoon until well blended. Cap the jar and leave it in a place free of drafts, direct sunlight, and extreme temperatures. Gently shake the jar once a day for 4 to 6 weeks, or until you feel that the fragrance has fully developed.

SWEET DREAMS

You can make this blend in larger quantities and sew it into herbal sleep pillows for a soothing effect. Stuff pillows and sachets with it, or set it out in a dish or bowl. You may use ¼ cup dill seed in place of the plant material.

> ½ cup chamomile flowers
> ½ cup sweet clover flowers
> ½ cup dill stems, leaves, and flowers
> ½ cup lavender flowers
> ½ cup sweet marjoram
> ¼ cup lemongrass or lemon balm leaves

Combine all ingredients in a glass jar and stir with a spoon until well blended. Cap the jar and leave it in a place free of drafts, direct sunlight, and extreme temperatures. Gently shake the jar once a day for 4 to 6 weeks, or until you feel that the fragrance has fully developed.

WINTER BLUES CHASER

This is a nice potpourri to have on hand for the winter holidays. I save plenty of needles from our Christmas tree and wreath each year, so I always have a supply of balsam, cedar, or pine available. The potpourri may be simmered in a pan of hot water on the stove, added to pillows and sachets, or set out in a dish or bowl.

> 1 cup evergreen needles
> ½ cup chopped dried apple
> ½ cup cedar chips
> ½ cup cinnamon sticks, broken into small pieces
> ¼ cup whole cloves
> 1 tablespoon allspice berries
> 1 tablespoon mace
> 1 tablespoon ground cinnamon
> 1 tablespoon chopped gingerroot
> 15 drops frankincense essential oil
> 10 drops myrrh essential oil

Combine all ingredients in a glass jar and stir with a spoon until well blended. Cap the jar and leave it in a place free of drafts, direct sunlight, and extreme temperatures. Gently shake the jar once a day for 4 to 6 weeks, or until you feel that the fragrance has fully developed.

HERBAL MISTS

It's really quite simple to have an herbal spray air freshener available for every room of your home. It's a lot of fun to create unique blends that help eliminate unpleasant odors while expressing the "real you."

As a bonus, some sprays can perform double duty. For instance, in the kitchen, a small spray bottle of distilled water and thyme essential oil can be used to tame pungent cooking odors and as a wash for fruits and vegetables. Spray the produce and gently scrub with a vegetable brush. Rinse well in clean water.

Decorative cobalt glass bottles are a great choice if the herbal mist will be in view. Of course, you can use almost any spray bottle or even a plant mister. Plastic bottles are a good choice for households with small children or animals; always be sure to keep the mixtures out of their reach.

To make your own herbal spray air freshener, first wash the container thoroughly. Then fill it with water (use distilled if it's also going to come in contact with human skin or foods; do not use the spray on skin within 12 hours of exposure to sun) and add 5 to 7 drops of an essential oil or combination of oils per 8 ounces of water. Here are some suggested blends:

- Country Spice — cinnamon, ginger, vanilla, bay
- Spring Morning — lavender, rose, geranium, rosemary, sweet orange

- Earthy — sage, thyme, cedar, patchouli, frankincense
- Romance — vanilla, sandalwood, ylang ylang, jasmine, neroli, rose
- Far East — patchouli, cedar, sandalwood, lime, coriander
- Energizing — basil, lavender, orange, nutmeg, mint
- Calming — bergamot, geranium, clary sage, chamomile, yarrow
- Gardener's Paradise — lemon, orange, basil, thyme

SIMPLE SACHETS

Sachets made from dried herbs and flowers will keep your linens and clothing smelling sweet while keeping insects at bay. A sachet formula doesn't need to be complicated to be effective — just a few ingredients are all that's required. In fact, if you don't have any dried herbs or flowers available, you can stuff the sachet with a bit of moss or even polyester fill scented with essential oil.

Sachets can be made in just minutes by stitching a double-layered square of cheesecloth, muslin, or a scrap of fabric on three sides and tying with a ribbon. You can also make use of those socks that mysteriously return mateless from the laundry room; socks are ideal for making sachets to scent sneakers, boots, and shoes.

These are some of my favorite ways to use sachets:

- Hang them in clothes closets or coat closets.
- Place them in dresser drawers.
- Use them to keep seasonal clothes fresh when being stored, such as in a trunk or storage closet.
- Put some in your sneakers, gardening shoes, or any other regularly used shoes.
- Tuck them under sheets and towels in the linen closet.

SWEET LINENS SACHET

This sachet recipe imparts a sweet aroma to linens and towels. Remember, all herbal materials should be dried before using in sachets. Depending on the size of the squares, this recipe will make four to six sachets.

> 4 cups oakmoss
> 2 cups rosemary leaves and flowers
> 2 cups lavender leaves and flowers
> ½ cup lemon balm or lemon verbena
> 1 tablespoon orrisroot
> 8 drops lavender essential oil
> 6 drops rosemary essential oil

Combine the dried herbs in a glass or ceramic bowl. Add the orrisroot and stir with a wooden spoon. Add the essential oils and mix well. Place spoonfuls of the blend onto muslin or cloth squares, leaving enough room to sew the sides together. Place sachets on shelves or hang inside linen closets and cupboards.

Spiced Sachets

This recipe has a zesty aroma and is especially nice to use around the holidays to scent linens for guests. You'll have enough filling for two to four sachets.

> 2 cups cinnamon chips
> ½ cup whole cloves
> ½ cup whole peppercorns
> ½ cup dried gingerroot slices
> 2 tablespoons ground cinnamon
> 1 tablespoon aniseed
> 2 teaspoon caraway seed

Combine all ingredients in a bowl and mix by hand or with a spoon to blend. Place spoonfuls of the blend onto muslin or cloth squares, leaving enough room to sew the sides together.

Deserving Drawers

This recipe is great to use in sock and sweater drawers. It lends a long-lasting earthy scent. Makes four to six sachets.

> 3 cups cedar chips
> 2 cups oakmoss
> 1 cup sandalwood chips
> 1 cup dried sage
> 1 vanilla bean, crushed
> 15 drops patchouli essential oil

Combine the cedar, oakmoss, sandalwood, and sage in a glass or ceramic bowl. Mix with a wooden spoon. Add the vanilla bean and patchouli oil and stir until completely mixed. Place spoonfuls of the blend onto muslin or cloth squares, leaving enough room to sew the sides together.

HERBAL SNEAKER TAMER #1

If your sneakers advertise the fact that you've been working hard, this recipe will help you keep the "news" to yourself.

  2 cups dried sage
1½ cups dried lemon balm
  2 cups cedar chips
  ½ cup baking soda
  2 tablespoons grated orange rind
 10 drops rosemary essential oil
  5 drops lemon essential oil

Combine the dried herbs, cedar chips, baking soda, and orange rind in a glass or ceramic bowl. Stir with a wooden spoon. Add the essential oils and stir to blend. Place half of the mixture in a clean sock and tie the open end shut. Stuff another sock with the remaining mixture and tie off. Place a stuffed sock in each sneaker overnight or when not in use.

HERBAL SNEAKER TAMER #2

Here's another odor-absorbing recipe to make your sneakers less unruly. Be sure to use only dried herbs in your potpourris.

  2 cups natural clay cat litter
  1 cup baking soda
  1 cup calendula flowers
  1 cup peppermint or spearmint leaves
  ½ cup thyme leaves
 10 drops peppermint essential oil
 10 drops wintergreen essential oil
 10 drops eucalyptus essential oil

Combine the cat litter and baking soda in a glass or ceramic bowl and mix with a wooden spoon. Add the herbs and mix again. Add the essential oils and blend. Place half of the mixture in each of two clean socks and tie the open ends shut. Place a stuffed sock in each sneaker overnight or when not in use.

MORE FRAGRANT IDEAS

Don't limit yourself to the three main types of air fresheners discussed here — be creative!

Hang dried herbs in closets and storage rooms to deter insects. Some good choices are mints, rosemary, lavender, sage, lemongrass, and citronella.

* * * * *

Place a few drops of essential oil on the outside of the filter bag of your vacuum cleaner.

* * * * *

If you have a fireplace, place two or three drops of essential oil of choice on the wood before lighting.

* * * * *

Add a few drops of a citrus essential oil to your humidifier. Do not use essential oils for this purpose if you suffer from asthma, however.

* * * * *

Add one or two drops of essential oil to the rings made to attach to the bulb of a standing lamp. The heat of the bulb will release the fragrance when the lamp is in use. Don't allow the essential oil to come in direct contact with the bulb; this can cause the bulb to explode and could result in a fire.

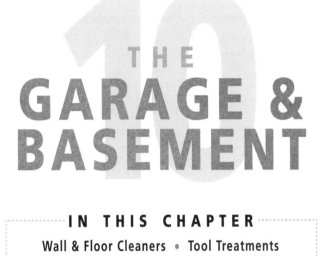

THE
GARAGE &
BASEMENT

Herbs and other natural materials can be used to clean up oil and grease spills in your basement or garage and to care for items stored in these areas, including tools and cars.

WALLS AND FLOORS

You may think it's silly to clean the walls and floors of a garage or basement, but these areas can take on unpleasant odors and invading pathogens such as mold and mildew. And if the garage or basement is used for recreation or work, you'll especially appreciate the removal of these unwelcome visitors. The following formulas are made from simple ingredients and they are as effective as they are easy to use.

OIL SPILL REMOVER

If you're fortunate enough to be able to park your car in the garage, then one thing is certain: You will have occasional oil leaks or spills on the garage floor. Try this simple trick to remove the oil and its telltale odor. Note: *Dry concrete mix can be used in place of the cat litter.*

    2 cups natural cat litter
    ½ cup baking soda
    8 drops eucalyptus or peppermint essential oil

Combine all ingredients in a small bucket or pail. Sprinkle mixture over the oil spill and let stand for 2 to 3 days. Then just sweep up the powder.

MOLD & MILDEW DESTROYER

This formula works well on concrete and walls made of cinder block. Try it out in your garage or your basement. Note: *A string mop works best on cinder block walls because their texture tends to tear sponge mop heads.*

    ½ gallon water
    2 cups hot vinegar
    1 cup lemon juice
    2 teaspoons tea tree essential oil

Combine all ingredients in a large bucket. Dip a mop into the bucket and wring out excess liquid. Wipe walls from the top down, rewetting the mop after a few strokes. Do not rinse. You can also wash concrete floors with this solution. If there are windows in the room, open them and let everything air-dry for a few hours.

CARING FOR TOOLS

To keep garden tools in good working order, they should be clean and dry before storing. Use a wire brush to remove dirt, and wipe tools with a dry cloth if they have any mud or moisture on them.

TOOL CONDITIONER

Large tools like shovels and rakes should be stored in this mixture to prevent rusting.

> 1 quart olive oil
> sand

Mix the olive oil into a bucket full of sand. Push large tools head first into the mixture and leave there when not in use.

Helpful Hints for Tool Maintenance

To clean any rusted tools, first rub with fine steel wool. Wipe with a rag moistened with a bit of olive oil before storing.

* * * * *

Peg board is a big tool-storing help in the garage. And if you outline your tools on the board with a pencil, you'll know when and what is missing.

* * * * *

Paint the handles of your tools a bright color, such as yellow or red. That way they'll be seen before they're stepped on or hit by the lawn mower.

* * * * *

Old tools can be recycled by turning them into garden ornaments. I use an old push broom handle to support a weather vane in one of my flower gardens. Antique tools can be displayed as a collection on the wall of a den or workshop. Just use your imagination!

CLEAN YOUR CAR NATURALLY

Even your automobiles can be cared for without the use of the toxic products currently sold for this purpose. The following formulas can be applied to your car, truck, boat, or recreational vehicle. Wear protective gloves when using these mixtures.

EASY CITRUS CAR WASH

This extremely simple formula is all you need to get your car clean.

- 1 gallon water
- ¼ cup liquid soap
- 10 drops lemon or orange essential oil

Fill a bucket with the water and liquid soap and stir until mixed. Add the essential oil and stir again. Using a soft cloth or sponge, wash the exterior of your car from the top down, one section at a time. Rinse each area well with clean water before the soap has a chance to dry.

GET-TOUGH-TO-GET-DIRT-GOING FORMULA

This formula is for added shine and to remove really tough dirt and grime.

> 1 gallon water
> ½ cup lemon juice
> 6 drops eucalyptus or mint essential oil
> ¼ cup liquid soap
> 3 tablespoons baking soda

Mix the water, lemon juice, essential oil, and liquid soap in a bucket. Add the baking soda and stir until blended. With a soft cloth or sponge, wash the exterior of your car from the top down, working in sections. Rinse each area well with clean water before the soap dries.

TIRE WASH

Use this cleaner to keep your tires looking like new.

> 2 cups baking soda
> ½ cup water
> ¼ cup liquid soap
> 2 cups vinegar or lemon juice
> 5 drops lemon, lime, or orange essential oil

Combine the baking soda, water, and soap in a bucket or other container. Add the vinegar and essential oil and mix well. Apply with a brush to get in between the tire treads. Wash one tire at a time, rinsing each before moving on to the next.

HEADLIGHT SCRUB

This formula will easily remove grime and the remains of insects that have met their end on your headlights.

> ¼ cup baking soda
> 1½ tablespoons liquid soap
> 8 drops eucalyptus or pine essential oil

Combine all ingredients in a plastic bowl and mix well. Dip a cloth, brush, or sponge into the wash and scrub each headlight. Rinse several times with a wet cloth or sponge or with a garden hose.

HERBAL CAR WAX

An all-natural recipe, this wax really protects your car's finish. It can be made in larger quantities and stored.

> 3 tablespoons beeswax
> 3 tablespoons carnauba wax
> 1 cup linseed oil
> 6 drops orange or lemon essential oil
> ½ cup lemon juice

1. Melt waxes and linseed oil together in a double boiler, stirring often. Add the essential oil, stir once and immediately remove from heat.

2. Pour the mixture into a clean coffee can. (*Careful:* The can will become hot.) Using gloves or potholders, place the coffee can in a place where it will be undisturbed for a few days.

3. When the wax has completely hardened, tap the sides out of the can until the wax breaks free. Turn out the wax and rub it directly on your car.

4. Dip a soft cloth into the lemon juice and squeeze dry. Polish the waxed car with the lemon juice–soaked cloth, then buff to a shine with a dry cloth.

FRESH-SCENT VINYL UPHOLSTERY CLEANER

If you're sensitive to that "new car smell," this formula will help eliminate it.

> 2 tablespoons baking soda
> 2 cups hot water
> 1 teaspoon orange, cedar, or mint
>   essential oil

Dissolve baking soda in hot water. Blend in essential oil. Vacuum the upholstery to remove loose dirt and debris from crevices and between the seats. (Watch out for loose change!) Moisten a soft cloth with the formula and rub over the upholstery, working from the top down. Rinse with a clean, damp cloth then dry to a shine with a dry towel.

LAVENDER LEATHER UPHOLSTERY CLEANER

To safely clean leather and impart a light lavender scent, try this formula. After cleaning, apply Fragrant Leather Uphol-stery Conditioner (page 153).

> ¼ cup soap flakes
> 1 cup hot water
> 6 drops mint or lavender essential oil

Dissolve soap flakes in hot water. Add essential oil and blend. Apply this formula with a soft brush, using gentle downward strokes. Wipe with a clean, damp cloth. Buff dry with a towel.

Old-Fashioned Cloth Upholstery Cleaner

This is an old-time recipe that really works!

> 2 cups water
> ¼ cup dried soapwort root *or* ¾ cup fresh
> stems

1. If using the dried root, soak it in the 2 cups of water overnight. If using fresh material, chop the stems into 1-inch pieces.

2. Bring the soapwort and water to a boil for 1 minute. Reduce heat and simmer for 20 minutes, stirring occasionally. Remove from heat and let the decoction stand until cool. Strain, and the cleaner is ready to use.

3. Dip a cloth or brush into the cleaner and rub into the upholstery using a downward motion. Rinse with a clean, damp cloth. Allow the upholstery to air-dry.

Fragrant Leather Upholstery Conditioner

Use this conditioner after cleaning your leather upholstery with Lavender Leather Upholstery Cleaner (page 152). The olive oil and rosemary tea will keep leather seats soft and conditioned.

> ½ cup olive oil
> ¼ cup strong rosemary tea
> ¼ cup vinegar

Combine all ingredients in a spray bottle and shake well. Lightly spray onto upholstery and buff with a dry cloth.

Quick Chrome Cleaner

If there are a lot of stains or bugs stuck on the chrome parts of your car, you can use a nylon-backed sponge with this formula. Make your own nylon sponge by securing a square of onion bag netting over a clean sponge or cloth. Note: Use a squirt-top bottle for this recipe, since the mixture may clog the nozzle of a spray bottle.

½ cup baking soda

¼ cup lemon juice

3 drops citrus essential oil of choice

Combine baking soda and lemon juice in a squirt bottle. Add the essential oil and shake well. Apply directly to chrome and wipe with a damp cloth. Rinse with clean water.

Dashboard Restorer

This simple formula will make your dashboard look brand new again.

1 cup water

½ cup vegetable oil–based soap (such as Murphy's Oil Soap)

10 drops cedar essential oil

Combine all ingredients in a small spray bottle and shake well. Spray onto dashboard and wipe clean with a soft cloth.

Window Wash

In the winter, this formula helps reduce frost buildup.

3 cups vinegar

1 cup water

10 drops lemon essential oil

Combine all ingredients in a large spray bottle and shake well. Spray liberally onto windows and wipe clean with a chamois cloth.

Tar Solvent

This formula is for those specks of tar that land on your car after driving on a freshly paved road.

> 1 tablespoon lemon juice or vinegar
> 2 teaspoons lemon essential oil
> 4 drops tea tree essential oil

Mix all ingredients in a small bowl. Rub some of the solution into tar with glove-protected fingertips or a sponge to loosen. Allow the formula to remain on the tar for 15 minutes, then wipe or scrape the remaining tar off with a nylon-backed sponge.

Mat & Carpet Cleaner and Deodorizer

Even if you've cleaned your car inside and out, dingy mats and carpeting will spoil the effect. This solution not only cleans the items, but also makes them smell fresh again.

> ½ gallon hot water
> ½ cup liquid soap
> 12 drops wintergreen or peppermint
>   essential oil

1. Combine all ingredients in a bucket or pail. Stir thoroughly to mix.

2. Vacuum loose dirt from carpeting and mats. Remove mats from the car and clean by dipping a brush into the cleaning solution and rubbing into the carpet fibers. Rinse the mats with a hose and allow them to dry in the sun.

3. Clean the carpeting on the floor of the car by dipping a brush into the cleaning solution and rubbing into the carpet. Wipe with a dry towel. Vacuum again when completely dry.

HERBAL FRAGRANCE POUCH

You also can make this air-freshening pouch with a single larger piece of fabric gathered at the top with a piece of colorful ribbon.

> 2 squares of fabric, 4 x 4 inches each
> 1 square of cotton batting, 3 x 3 inches, *or* six cotton balls
> 5 drops cedar essential oil
> 5 drops patchouli essential oil
> 3 drops sandalwood essential oil
> 2 drops neroli (orange blossom) or sweet orange essential oil

1. Place one of the squares of fabric on a flat surface, pattern side down. On top of this place the cotton batting or cotton balls. Add the essential oils to the cotton and place the remaining square of fabric, pattern side up, on top.

2. Stitch or use a hot glue gun to seal the edges of the fabric squares. Attach a loop or strand of ribbon at the top and hang it from your rearview mirror.

Instant Herbal Car Deodorizer

If your pets frequently travel in the car, then you know how odors can linger long after the ride is over. This formula will eliminate those odors.

>   ¾ cup water
>   ¼ cup vinegar
>   6 drops lavender essential oil
>   4 drops lemon essential oil
>   4 drops sweet orange essential oil
>   2 drops peppermint essential oil

Combine all ingredients in a small spray bottle (about 8 ounces) and shake well. Hold the spray bottle 6–8 inches from surfaces and lightly mist upholstery and carpeting. Leave the windows and doors open for 15 minutes after spraying, if possible. Don't let Fido back into the car immediately, as the essential oils can irritate his paws and sensitive nose.

EMERGENCY CARE FOR MOTION SICKNESS

If someone in your family is prone to carsickness, you don't want to be without this simple remedy! Place 2 or 3 drops of peppermint *or* ginger essential oil on a tissue. Sniff the tissue until the feeling passes. Although this treatment usually works well for people, I can't be sure about its effect on the family dog.

FRUITY TRAVEL WIPES

These travel wipes are quick and easy to make. They sure come in handy too!

- 10 drops lemon essential oil
- 4 drops grapefruit seed extract
- 6 drops lime essential oil
- 2 drops tea tree essential oil
- 10 squares cut from cellulose sponge cloth or cotton T-shirts, 5 x 8 inches each

1. Fold each square of cloth in half and place in a plastic zipper bag or a small plastic container with an airtight lid. Add enough water to saturate each cloth, but not enough to cover them.

2. Press down on the cloths with one hand and drain excess water into a cup. Add the remaining ingredients to the water and stir. Pour this mixture over the cloths once more and seal the container.

3. Keep in the glove compartment of your car and use when needed to clean hands and face.

SUDDEN SPILL & SPOT REMOVER

It never fails — someone spills ice cream or soda on the floor or upholstery just as you've pulled onto the highway. This formula will lift out most stains, including those left by greasy foods, and leave a fresh, clean smell.

- ½ cup vinegar
- ½ cup club soda
- 8 drops eucalyptus essential oil
- 3 drops wintergreen essential oil

Combine all ingredients in a small spray bottle and shake well. Spray directly onto stain and blot with a clean, dry cloth. Repeat as necessary.

UNDER-THE-HOOD MAINTENANCE

You didn't think you'd see any herbal formulas in this department, did you? In truth, there aren't many, but what is presented here is useful nonetheless. These formulas can be used on the engine of your car, lawn mower, or other machinery.

ENGINE DEGREASER

A buildup of oil and grease on an engine can adversely affect performance, and could result in engine fire. Cut through grease with this powerful cleaner.

> ¼ cup washing soda
> 1 cup water
> 1 cup vinegar
> 25 drops tea tree essential oil
> 20 drops citrus essential oil of choice

1. Pour the washing soda into a plastic jug or pitcher, one with a tight-fitting cap and preferably a pour spout.

2. Bring the water and vinegar to a boil in a saucepan. Remove from heat and add to the pitcher. Cap the pitcher and shake to dissolve the washing soda. (*Careful* — it will be hot!) Add the essential oils and shake once more.

3. Slowly pour the solution over a *cool* engine (one that has not been run for at least an hour). Use a stiff brush to loosen oil and grease. Rinse with a garden hose or pour clean water over the engine several times. Leave the engine exposed to the air until completely dry.

RADIATOR RESCUE

This is a two-part formula. Use the wash for the exterior of your car radiator, then follow with the finishing treatment to deter rust.

Wash:

>2 cups boiling water
>¾ cup washing soda
>6 drops rosemary essential oil

Finish:

>1 cup water
>2 teaspoons pure linseed oil

1. Combine wash ingredients in a bowl or other container; stir to mix. Pour over a *cool* radiator and use a brush to clean off any oil or grease residue.

2. Rinse with clean water and allow the radiator to air-dry.

3. Combine the finish ingredients in a small spray bottle and shake well. Lightly spray radiator. Allow to air-dry before using the vehicle.

GASKET & HOSE MAINTENANCE

A thin coating of olive oil applied to hoses and gaskets helps prevent cracking caused by exposure to extreme temperatures. Don't forget about the rubber seals around car doors. Pour a few tablespoons of olive oil into a cup, then dip the tip of a small paintbrush brush into the olive oil and shake off any excess. Apply the olive oil to rubber hoses, gaskets, and door seals. Go over these areas again with a dry cloth to remove excess oil.

BATTERY TERMINAL CLEANER

Battery terminals can develop a lot of gunk over time, leading to corrosion and a shortened life for your battery.

>   ½ cup baking soda
>   4 drops lime or orange essential oil
>   water to make a paste

Combine all ingredients in a small bowl or cup and blend well, using only enough water to make a paste of medium thickness. Apply the paste to battery terminals with an old toothbrush and scrub until clean. Wipe the terminals clean with a slightly damp cloth, then wipe again with a dry cloth.

CORROSION RESISTANCE FOR BATTERY TERMINALS

To keep unsightly battery corrosion from happening, use this simple formula. Note: The paintbrush you use can be restored by soaking it in hot vinegar.

>   ½ tablespoon 100% pure aloe vera gel
>   1 tablespoon petroleum jelly

Mix the aloe vera gel and petroleum jelly together in a cup. Apply the mixture to the battery terminals with the tip of a small paintbrush.

RESOURCES

Essential Oils and Dried Herbs

These companies sell essential oils, dried herbs and herbalist supplies such as droppers, glassware, labels, bags and more.

Aphrodisia
282 Bleecker Street
New York, NY 10014
(212) 989-6440

Aroma Vera
5901 Rodeo Road
Los Angeles, CA 90016-4312
(800) 669-9514

Church Hill Herbs
608 Chimborazo
 Boulevard
Richmond, VA 23223
(888) 431-7627

The Essential Oil Company
P.O. Box 206
Lake Oswego, OR 97034
(800) 729-5912

Frontier Herbs
2264 Market Street
San Francisco, CA 94114
(800) 786-1388

Goodwin Creek Gardens
P.O. Box 83
Williams, OR 97544
(541) 846-7357

Monarda Herbal Apothecary
P.O. Box 505
Rosendale, NY 12472
(914) 658-7044

Mountain Rose
20818 High Street
North San Juan, CA
 95960
(800) 879-3337

Nature's Herb Company
1010 Forty-Sixth Street
Emeryville, CA 94608
(415) 601-0700

Summer's Past Farms
15602 Old Highway 80
El Cajon, CA 92021
(800) 340-9969

Herb Farms and Nurseries

These companies offer seeds and plants for your garden.

Blossom Farm
34515 Capel
Columbia Station, OH
  44028

The Herb Farm
32804 Issaquah-Fall City
  Road
Fall City, WA 98024
(206) 784-2222
Web site: www.theherb-
  farm.com

Ladybug Herbs
RR1, Box 3380
Wolcott, VT 05680
(802) 888-5940

Nichols Garden Nursery
1190 NE Pacific
Albany, OR 97321
(541) 928-9280

Sunnyboy Gardens
3314 Earlysville Road
Earlysville, VA 22936
(804) 974-7350
Web site: www.sunny-
  boygardens.com

Well-Sweep Herb Farm
205 Mount Bethel Road
Port Murray, NJ 07865
(908) 852-5390

Nontoxic Cleaning Supplies

The following is a list of mail-order suppliers that distribute safe cleaning products and supplies. Many have catalogs available; call or write to request one.

Allergy Resources, Inc.
557 Burbank Street,
  Suite K
Broomfield, CO 80020
(800) 873-3529

Auro Organics
Sinan Company
P.O. Box 857
Davis, CA 95617-0857
(916) 753-3104

Automation, Inc.
11232-1 St. John's
  Industrial Parkway
Jacksonville, FL 32246
(904) 998-9888

Desert Essence
9510 Vassar Avenue,
  Unit A
Chatsworth, CA 91311
(818) 709-8525

Dr. Bronner's
All-One-God Faith, Inc.
P.O. Box 28
Escondido, CA 92033

Earth Tribe
3303 Pico Boulevard
Santa Monica, CA
  90405
(800) 887-4238
Web site: www.earth-
  tribe.com

Ecco Bella
125 Tompton Plains
  Crossroads
Wayne, NJ 07479

Eco-House, Inc.
P.O. Box 220, Station A
Fredericton, New
  Brunswick
E3B 4Y9 Canada

Harmony Catalog
360 Interlocken
  Boulevard, Suite 300
Broomfield, CO 80021
(800) 456-1177
Web site: www.har-
  monycatalog.com

Life on the Planet
23852 Pacific Coast
  Highway #200
Malibu, CA 90265
(818) 880-5144

Life Tree Products
A Division of Sierra
  Dawn
P.O. Box 1203
Sebastopol, CA 95472
(707) 577-0324

Naturally Yours
Ecolo-International, Ltd.
717 North West Bypass
Springfield, MO 65802
(417) 865-6260

Seventh Generation
49 The Meadow Park
Colchester, VT 05446
(800) 456-1177

Watkins
150 Liberty Street
P.O. Box 5570
Winona, MN 55987-
0570
(360) 671-1672
Web site: www.dlban-
ning.com/html/home-
care.html

Safe Pet Products
**The Natural Pet
Care Catalog**
8050 Lake City Way
Seattle, WA 98115
(800) 962-8266
Web site: www.all-the-
best.com

**Nature's Earth
Products**
2200 North Florida
Mango Road, 2nd
Floor
West Palm Beach, FL
33409
(800) 749-PINE
Web site: www.natures-
earth.com
Organic cat litter

**North Star Natural
Pet Products**
148 Channel Road
Tinmouth, VT 05773
(802) 446-2812

**P.O.R.G.I.E. Natural
Pet Supply**
2023 Chicago Avenue,
Suite B22
Riverside, CA 92507-
2311
(888) 2-PORGIE

INDEX

Page numbers in *italics* indicate charts.

OTHER STOREY TITLES
YOU WILL ENJOY

The Aromatherapy Companion, by Victoria H. Edwards.
Prominent aromatherapist Edwards has created the most compre-
hensive aromatherapy guide available. Readers will find detailed
profiles of dozens of essential oils, instructions for blending and
using them, and information on aromatherapy for the different
stages of life. 288 pages. Paperback. ISBN 1-58017-150-8.

Creating Fairy Garden Fragrances, by Linda K. Gannon. This
beautifully illustrated book explores the magical, aromatic world of
herbs and flowers and provides recipes for richly scented, exotic potpourri blends. Aside each blend are fairy and herbal lore, poetry, sto-
ries about the seasons and the enchanted creatures of the garden, and
gift packaging ideas. 64 pages. Hardcover. ISBN 1-58017-076-5.

The Essential Oils Book, by Colleen K. Dodt. A rich resource on
the many applications of aromatherapy and its uses in everyday life,
this book includes aromas for the home, office, and essences for the
elderly. 160 pages. Paperback. ISBN 0-88266-913-3.

Keeping Life Simple, by Karen Levine. This easy-to-read book
helps readers assess what's really satisfying and then offers hundreds
of tips for creating a lifestyle that is more rewarding. 160 pages.
Paperback. ISBN 0-88266-943-5.

The Stain and Spot Remover Handbook, by Jean Cooper.
Everything you need to know to remove unsightly blemishes in a
single, easy-to-use reference. This book explains how to treat stains
caused by different sources and how to avoid making a problem
worse. 160 pages. Paperback. ISBN 0-88266-811-0.

Too Busy to Clean?, by Patti Barrett. This witty, realistic handbook
is filled with shortcuts and tricks for making cleaning more tolerable
and efficient. Also included are tips for getting organized and cleaning just about anything. 160 pages. Paperback. ISBN 1-58017-029-3.

Unclutter Your Home, by Donna Smallin. This books offers hundreds of steps for sorting, evaluating, and getting rid of all those
material items that get in the way of a simplified life. Learn how to
clean out every corner of your living space and create a more peace-
ful environment. 192 pages. Paperback. ISBN 1-58017-108-7.

These books and other Storey books are available at your bookstore,
farm store, garden center, or directly from Storey Books, Schoolhouse
Road, Pownal, Vermont 05261, or by calling 1-800-441-5700.
Or visit our Web site at www.storeybooks.com.